Dedicated to all of the volunteers and individuals in HealingStrong™ who are serving their communities, leading HealingStrong groups, and helping people find true Hope.

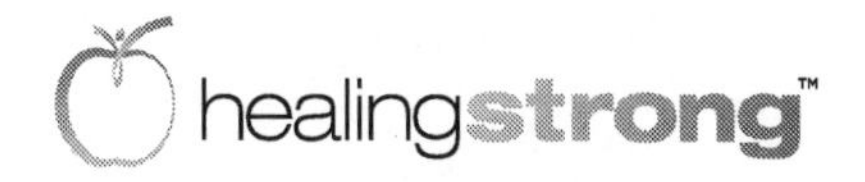

Suzy Griswold, MPH
Founder, HealingStrong™

Mary
404 823 4257

Lindsey
770-865-4135

Disclaimer:
The content of this document is based on research conducted by the author. The information is presented for educational purposes only and is not intended to diagnose or prescribe for any medical or psychological condition, nor to prevent, treat, mitigate or cure such conditions. The information contained herein is not intended to replace a one-on-one relationship with a doctor or qualified healthcare professional. It is not intended as medical advice, but rather a sharing of knowledge and information based on personal research and experience. HealingStrong™ encourages you to make your own health care decisions based on your own judgment and research in partnership with a qualified healthcare professional. These statements have not been evaluated by the Food and Drug Administration.

100% of donations raised from downloads of this e-book will support the growth and expansion of HealingStrong™ Groups around the world.

"This book is dedicated to my family members who died from cancer never knowing about alternative treatment therapies."

Alfred Presnell, Pat O'Brien-Presnell,
Gloria Presnell-Mosher, Grace Robinson,
Evelyn Gardner, Toni Sue Cave, Mike O'Brien,
Robert O'Brien, Bobbie O'Brien-Gardner,
and Connie O'Brien.

Please help us to get the word out to others. Share our website:
www.healingstrong.org
and our Facebook Page
www.facebook.com/healingstrong
with your friends and family.

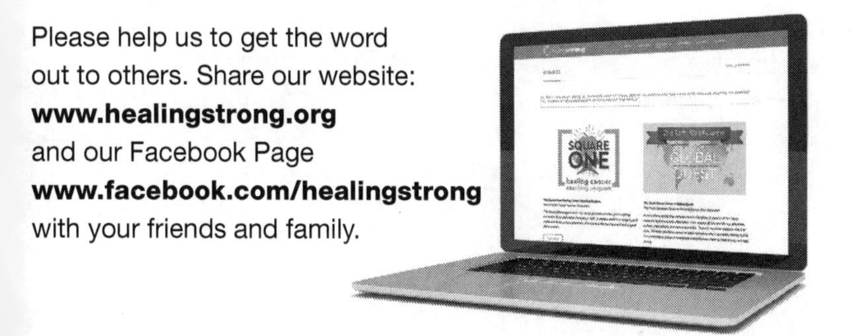

FOREWORD

Suzy and I met in a grocery store coffee shop in the spring of 2013, to share our personal healing journeys. She had been healed of thyroid cancer and I had healed from breast cancer, outside of traditional medicine. I immediately "fell in love" with Suzy and her passion to share her Aha! Moments with the world. When we met, I could sense her zeal and excitement. Suzy was on a mission to serve and to guide people who were diagnosed with cancer, but needed support and education about evidence-based natural medicine.

When I felt that fateful lump in my left breast, I had been in practice as a bio-energetic chiropractor for 25 years. Although I had seen amazing changes in my patients, now it was time for me to experience my own healing journey. I found myself frustrated, confused and even overwhelmed at times because of all the information out there. I was alone and I did not have a support group that understood why I was not addressing breast cancer using the traditional medical model of chemo, surgery and radiation.

So when I heard Suzy's mission about HealingStrong™, it was for me, an "Aha! Moment". I was so impressed with her clarity and desire to share hope with others, that I became one of the speakers for the first HealingStrong™ conference; and afterwards, joined together with a small group of cancer survivors to start the very first HealingStrong™ group. It has been four short years since then, and HealingStrong™ groups are educating and empowering communities in the United States, Canada, South Africa, and South Australia. Suzy's Aha! Moments have turned into a grassroots movement helping thousands of people connect truths about healing.

The testimonials speak for themselves. With proper guidance, a balanced diet and a change in lifestyle, the body has the ability to regain vibrant health. As Suzy mentions, "cancer is a process, not a thing."

The medical model for treating cancer is broken. Traditional medical doctors are not educating their patients about the powerful healing mechanisms of the body. They look at "the cancer" as the problem, without addressing the whole person – physical, mental, spiritual and emotional.

HealingStrong™ understands the pillars of health and what it takes to reverse cancer. The curriculum, the information provided, the support and the spiritual connection, provide a harmonious and loving touch to a very distressing situation – a cancer diagnosis.

A cancer diagnosis changes your life forever. By applying the principles provided by the HealingStrong™ support groups, that journey becomes less fearful and charged with hope. This book offers the person with little or no knowledge of holistic health a starting point of understanding. It is a powerful tool of hope.

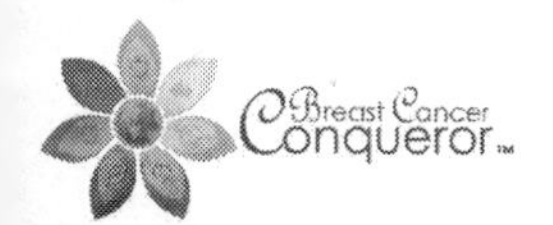

Dr. Véronique Desaulniers
Breast Cancer Conqueror

TABLE OF CONTENTS

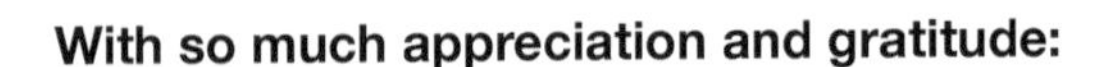

With so much appreciation and gratitude:

Bailey Bowe & Donna Brady, Testimonial Editors

Linda Perkins, Editor
lindawperkins.com

Homer Carvajal – Carvajal Creative
Print Layout and Design
carvajalcreative.com

"We should be paying more attention to the exceptional patients, those who get well unexpectedly, instead of staring bleakly at all those who die in the usual pattern. In the words of Rene' Dubos, sometimes the more measurable drives out the most important."

Bernie B.Siegel, M.D.,
in *Love, Medicine and Miracles*

PREFACE

I have learned through the course of my career and personal journey of healing my own cancer that doctors are limited by the American Medical Association and Federal Drug Administration on what they can do to treat cancer. As a matter of fact, treatment of cancer in the United States by medical doctors is accomplished in one of three ways: surgery, radiation or chemotherapy. Anything else prescribed by doctors may open them up to lawsuits and even loss of their license to practice medicine.

In light of the above, I first want to say that my goal is not to put down the medical establishment. Many medical conditions that would have been a death sentence 50 years ago are now easily cured with the advancements in medicine. However, while these advancements have made a significant impact on other diseases and health problems, cancer is different. I am here to tell you what I have learned in my own journey to healing that was not readily available to me in my doctors' offices.

The first time I ever heard about cancer, I was just five years old. My mom would not allow me to spend the night with a friend because her dad had "cancer." She was afraid of the disease, what it was

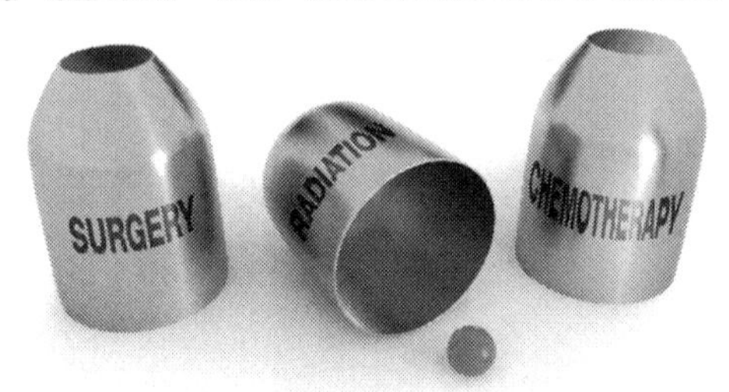

doing to my friend's father, and most of all, she was afraid I could somehow "get it" – as if it was some kind of infectious disease like polio. You see, in 1972, cancer was almost unheard of. It wasn't fully understood at the time.

The irony in the story is that not long after that, my Uncle Alfred died of pancreatic cancer. Thus began many years of my family's experience with cancer and the treatments that my loved ones endured. In all, ten of twelve family members who were diagnosed with cancer died, including my beloved mother. The deadly effect of cancer on my family significantly impacted me and my career choices.

In 1997, when I was a graduate student working on my Masters in Public Health at the University of Texas Health Science Center in Houston, I interned at a cancer foundation as a research coordinator. We were studying a cancer drug that was designated for pancreatic cancer patients, and it was showing great promise. We had one patient who did so well on this drug that his advanced, stage 4 pancreatic cancer was in "remission" and the tumor masses previously measurable were barely evident on the scans.

By the time I had joined the team, this patient (we'll call him Gordy) had been a part of the study for a while, and Gordy and his wife had become somewhat of a celebrity in the clinic. He was the "poster child" for the foundation and it was quite remarkable the outcome he was experiencing while on this drug. Well, I'll never forget a conversation I had with Gordy and his wife one day.

Gordy's wife pulled me aside during their routine "check-up" and asked me if I would like to know what they were doing besides the clinical trial drug. I said "of course". Her secret was a "macrobiotic diet": lots of lentils, vegetables, brown rice, no meat, no dairy, and no dessert. "Really?" I asked. Embarrassingly, I had no clue what she was talking about.

Yes, I was in graduate school at one of the largest health science centers in the world, and I sat there with a blank stare wondering to myself, "What did she just say?" I thought it was so odd and while I gave it no thought in relation to whether or not it had any impact on Gordy's success with the treatment, it did sit strong in my memory bank.

Fast forward many years, Gordy's story and the brief conversation that day came rushing back to me when I began to question traditional medicine after my own cancer diagnosis in 2009. I never spoke with Gordy or his wife again. Recently, with the help of the Internet, I went looking for Gordy and his wife. Unfortunately, he had passed away, having lived for 17 more years giving back to the community after surviving stage 4 advanced metastatic pancreatic cancer. I now know that their little secret had everything to do with Gordy's unexpectedly long life.

I have written in these pages the information that gripped me in a way I will never forget. It changed the way I looked at cancer, and ultimately the way I treated it after my own diagnosis. I have presented the information in a manner that is simple and to the point... just the way I like it.

I am not an expert on cancer or treatments, but I have had some pretty astounding "Aha! Moments" during my personal journey with cancer. They led me to make some drastic decisions on my course of treatments, and ultimately to start the HealingStrong™ organization.

These were important questions in my mind that I needed to resolve.

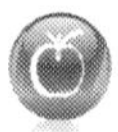

How is it that natural, non-toxic "alternative" therapies can be considered a viable option when my doctor doesn't even talk about them?

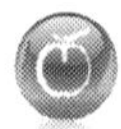

How in the world could I ever walk away from what my doctor is recommending? After all, he's the doctor.

These Aha! Moments were originally published on HealingStrong's™ very first website in 2012. Our website has changed quite a bit since then, but I still believe this information is useful. I hope that

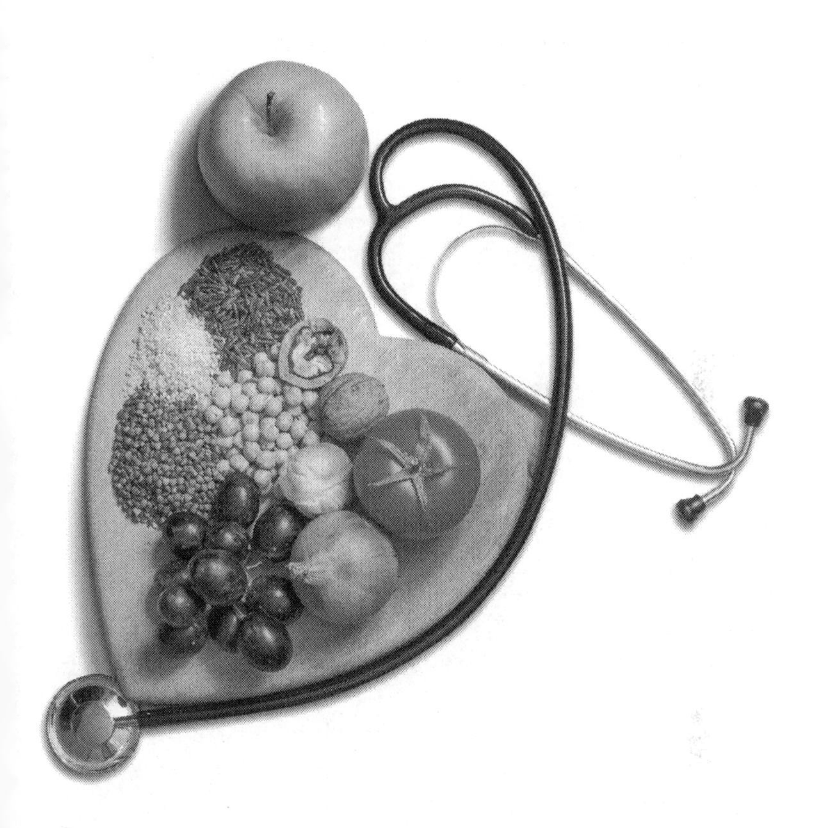

sharing it will give clarity to the questions that so many people have when faced with a cancer diagnosis, or when a well-meaning friend or family member is telling us to look into “alternative therapies.”

I hope and pray that you will find nuggets in this little book that will help you, your friend, or your loved one to begin to really grasp the bigger picture, and empower a decision that is not based on fear or lack of knowledge. A wonderful proverb reminds us of this:

“Wisdom is the principal thing; therefore get wisdom:
and with all thy getting get understanding.”

– **Proverbs 4:7** (KJV)

SUZY'S HEALING STRONG JOURNEY

My healing strong journey began in 2000 when a diagnosis of thyroid cancer stopped me in my tracks. I was already preparing to have surgery for a different health issue, so the diagnosis of cancer took me by surprise.

My healthcare providers made it seem like treating cancer in the thyroid gland was supposed to be a piece of cake. I was told many times that if you are going to get cancer, thyroid cancer is the cancer to get because it often responds well to radiation treatment. I had no reason not to trust them. I was already relying on multiple doctors and subsequently many prescription drugs for various health issues: insomnia, neck tremors, thyroid disease, and fibroid tumors. Now I would trust them with my cancer.

After undergoing thyroid surgery and radiation therapy, my next scan showed three glands "lit up". Discussions of radical neck dissection, plucking the lymph nodes "one by one", combination chemotherapy and more radiation ensued. They were all possibilities in my future. The doctors seemed okay with that — but I wasn't. My family's history and my personal experience with their deaths led me to explore other things.

In the meantime, a friend sent me a book by Suzanne Somers called Knockout. It profiled what medical doctors around the world were doing to diagnose and treat cancer – and it wasn't conventional. This book opened my eyes to the possibilities that I never was exposed to with my family members who had died of cancer. I often thought about them and wondered what they would think about this information. Would they believe it? If they would have tried these things, would they be here today?

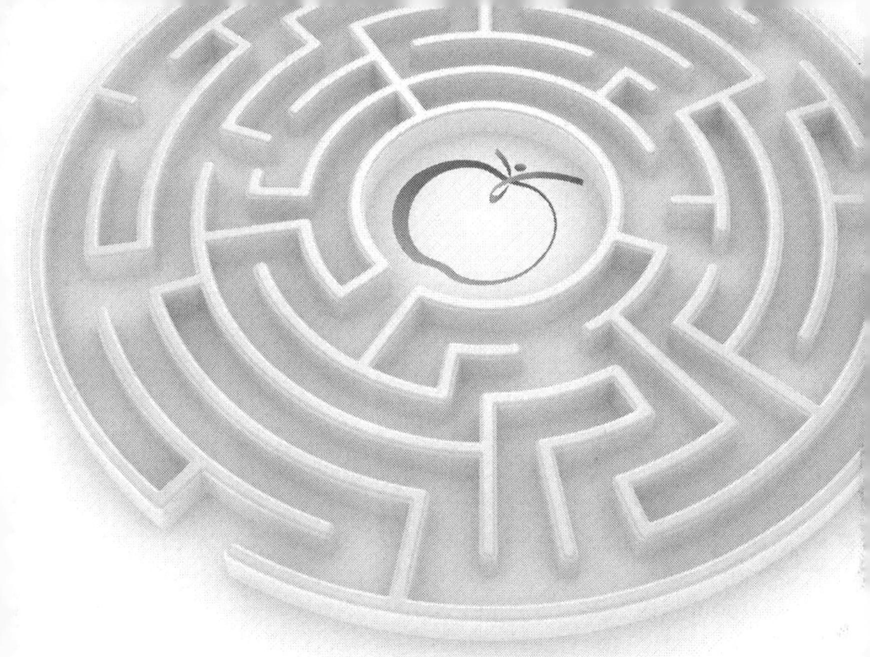

I continued to research alternative cancer treatments, including the science and history of cancer and epidemiological trends, and the work of Dr. Max Gerson made the most sense to me. Ultimately, I walked away from any further conventional treatment. Inspired most by Dr. Max Gerson and Anne Fraham, I committed to an extensive protocol that involved a vegan diet, juicing 8-10 juices a day, two to three coffee enemas a day, a regimen of supplements, reduced stress, rest, meditating and praying on God's healing words.

I even started selling natural soaps to my friends to help orphans in Africa have clean water. My 80+ year old friend and sister in Christ, Mary G., told me that a way to keep my mind uplifted was to help others. Jeff and our two boys committed to turning our home and our life into a healing place for a healing season.

It took about a year and a half of commitment to this lifestyle, but everything in my body healed –from the inside out. The cancer was gone, and my body was stronger than ever.

Make no mistake – I didn't walk away from the doctors' recommendations lightly. My husband was in a constant state of defense. Some in our church family and even long-time friends called him, expressing their concern and asking him to help me reconsider my decision for treatment. Especially in the beginning, he was also very fearful, but he committed to listening to the audio tapes, videos, and book excerpts that I would read to him late into the night.

In addition to my research, one of the reasons I was able to walk out my healing with confidence was that I sought out the success stories of those who incorporated holistic therapies into their protocol. I learned what the patients who were given the least hope did – how they fared using holistic therapies. I searched for their numbers online, called or emailed the ones I could reach.

Some of these cancer survivors' stories are included in this book. After my healing was complete, I invited those people who had impacted me throughout my journey to come together and we threw the biggest party ever: ***2013 HealingStrong™ Conference and Retreat***. Chris Wark, Dr. Linda Isaacs, Dr. Veronique Desaulniers, Ty Bollinger, Fr. John and Cherie Calbom, Robert Scott Bell, Dr. Judy Seeger, Dr. Kate Cirillo, Cortney Campbell, Wendy Hood, and others came together to share their stories of hope. Out of this conference birthed a mission and an organization, HealingStrong™.

Today, HealingStrong™ is growing in cities around the globe, helping people find hope, connection and encouragement through local community groups, led by those who have used holistic healing strategies in their own lives. My prayer is that whoever reads this book will discover truth and be led on a journey to healing from cancer or any disease with confidence and faith. Fear will be a thing of the past and your life will be lived with purpose and full of hope.

May the God of hope fill you with all joy and peace as you trust in him, so that you may overflow with hope by the power of the Holy Spirit.
Romans 15:13

"I shall not die, but live, and declare the works of the Lord."
Psalms 118:17

Aha! Moment #1
True Healing is Holistic

SUZY'S PERSONAL PERSPECTIVE

From the beginning, I didn't have a peace about the conventional therapies that were being discussed for my cancer treatment: "radical neck dissection," "pluck my glands out one by one," and chemotherapy. Part of this was due to the history of my family and cancer treatments, but I also just couldn't shake the uneasiness that I felt.

Eight months after my original diagnosis, I found myself in a very prominent and well-known doctor's office and he was telling me that I needed to do several months of chemotherapy. This didn't sit well with me, but I didn't know what else was out there.

In my mind, unconventional medicine or "alternative therapies" were things like "blood-letting", leaching, and recent discoveries, like "coffee enemas". That would be a great big "no" in my mind, but I owed it to myself to figure out if giving up my fried chicken, Starbucks coffee, and chocolate cake would make a difference. How in the world could that help me heal my cancer?

I began my research diving into the historical documents of medicine, starting with the Bible.

One of the first things I did in my research after being confronted with "alternative therapies as an option" was to examine the history of medicine in general.

First, I wanted to know what God's word says about "medicine" – because after all, I believe that He is the Living God and Creator of the Universe and His plans for me are good.

The true origins of medicine started when Adam and Eve were created. I had never read the Bible with glasses to see what God said about healing medicine. Well, the Bible is clear about the original intent of what we should eat and what we should use for healing. I ran across these scripts that I had read before, but this time – in light of where I was, it was different:

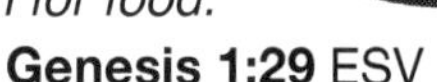

And God said, "Behold, I have given you every plant yielding seed that is on the face of all the earth, and every tree with seed in its fruit. You shall have them for food.

Genesis 1:29 ESV

Then the angel showed me the river of the water of life, bright as crystal, flowing from the throne of God and of the Lamb through the middle of the street of the city; also, on either side of the river, the tree of life with its twelve kinds of fruit, yielding its fruit each month. The leaves of the tree were for the healing of the nations.

Revelation 22:1-2 ESV

And to every beast of the earth and to every bird of the heavens and to everything that creeps on the earth, everything that has the breath of life, I have given every green plant for food." And it was so.

Genesis 1:30 ESV

He causeth the grass to grow for the cattle, and herb for the service of man: that he may bring forth food out of the earth.

Psalms 104:14-15

Starting in Genesis, and continuing through the old and new testaments, there are wonderful scriptures and stories about food helping to sustain and heal (dates and raisins packed to sustain during long trips, figs placed on boils to heal, and so much more).

Frankincense and myrrh were two important oils that I equated with the birth of Jesus, but I always was taught those were just "symbolic" for purification and Jesus' coming burial. I had an epiphany one day about the two oils mentioned in the manger scene. Would God require Mary to carry around large amounts of items as a "symbol"… or, was God himself providing the greatest medicine for a new mother who would be living out the infant days of her new baby Jesus in caves and sheep stalls? We knew gold was valuable and useful for living, but what about frankincense and myrrh? Well, the historical use of these two oils was quite useful, including wound care, analgesic, incense, antiseptic and many more uses.

Comparing the biblical text with recent scientific studies, I found in researching the national database on cancer research, PubMed, that there are 90 articles about the anti-tumor effect of frankincense, the resin extract from the Boswellia species. It has been used for treating various diseases with very minimal side effects, including all kinds of cancer.

Searching through the scriptures made me ask important questions that began to resonate in my heart. This began a snowball effect, as I looked into other natural cancer fighting herbs, such as curcumin or cinnamon (which helps to prevent angiogenesis in cancer, and therefore helps prevent it from spreading). I wanted to know more.

Scriptures were also very revealing in terms of our emotions, bitterness, unforgiveness affecting my health. Really? The fact that I harbored unforgiveness, bitterness and resentment in my heart could be a factor in my healing? The Living Word of God has something to say about it as you'll see in these verses from Proverbs:

A peaceful heart leads to a healthy body;
jealousy is like cancer in the bones.

Proverbs 14:30 NLT

A joyful heart is good medicine, but a crushed spirit dries up the bones. **Proverbs 17:22** ESV

These were important messages and I believe very literally what the Bible says is truth. I recently read a book titled You Can Beat the Odds by Brenda Stockdale. She started one of the book's sections out with Proverbs 17:22 (as mentioned on previous page). Then she goes on to present a very compelling study where a doctor out of Tampa Florida, David Vesely, Chief Endocrinologist at Veterans Hospital in Tampa and professor of medicine and pharmacology and physiology at the University of South Florida, examined heart hormones in vitro and their effect on cancer cells.

Vesley's study showed that heart hormones eliminated 97 percent of all cancer cells within only twenty-four hours. In mice, the same experiment yielded 80 percent elimination of pancreatic cancer and 66 percent of breast cancer was eliminated. The bottom line is that our body parts are so entwined and with the hormones in our heart tied to overall health, a joyful heart is very literally good medicine.

I kept searching scriptures for promises in His word, but also desired to examine the history in terms of medicine. During my college studies, as well as a short stint as an immunization program coordinator based out of a medical school, I studied Hippocrates. Hippocrates is considered the father of modern medicine and physicians take the Hippocratic Oath before leaving their formal medical studies and entering into "the real world" of mainstream medicine.

Some of his most famous sayings of his included:

"Let medicine be thy food, and food be thy medicine."

- Hippocrates

"Leave your drugs in the chemist's pot if you can heal the patient with food."

- Hippocrates

Wait! When did things change? If Hippocrates recognized food as healing, and other holistic healing as valid, why do my doctors call "alternative therapies" hog-wash?

Why is food the last thing doctors want to talk about when it comes to cancer? When my mother was dying of cancer, the doctors told my Dad and I to feed her milkshakes, Jell-O, whatever she would eat. So, we did... giving her lots of milkshakes. When I began to look at the history of medicine and put two and two together, my Aha! Moment came when I realized what doctors are taught in medical schools are centered around pharmacology, and limited in nutrition and its impact on disease.

I went back and read the Hippocratic Oath. It's quite revealing.

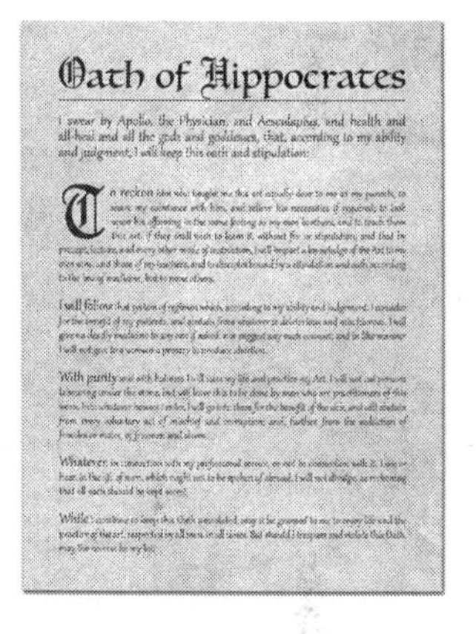

Oath of Hippocrates

I swear by Apollo the Physician, and Aesculapius, and health and all-heal and all the gods and goddesses, that, according to my ability and judgment, I will keep this oath and stipulation:

Today, there are lots of "modern versions" of the Oath that are interesting. For me, getting back to the basics was important. Reading the original Oath and studying some of Hippocrates practices and sayings impacted my Aha! Moment in this area. Today, physicians' approach of food as medicine is not the norm. I learned the following about current medical practices:

- Only 6% of physicians study nutrition in medical school. (Dr. Ray Strand, What Your Doctor Doesn't Know About Nutrition May Be Killing You, 2002)

- The current 23.9 hours of nutrition education training falls short of the NAS 1985 minimum recommendation and far short of the American Society for Clinical Nutrition (ASCN) 1989 recommendations. The ASCN recommendations were based on a survey of curriculum administrators and nutrition educators; the former group suggested 37 hours (median: 32), whereas the latter suggested 44 hours (median: 40) be devoted to nutrition instruction (9). Am J Clin Nutr. 1989 Oct;50(4):707-12. Priorities for nutrition content in a medical school curriculum: a national consensus of medical educators. Weinsier RL1, Boker JR, Brooks CM, Kushner RF, Visek WJ, Mark DA, Lopez-S A, Anderson MS, Block K.

This is contrary to the very Hippocratic Oath that has driven medicine for centuries. Hippocrates and his followers vowed to apply dietetic measures for the benefit of the sick; and to neither give a deadly drug to anybody who asked for it, nor make a suggestion to this effect.

Homeopathic practices (natural approaches to healing) were deemed highly successful through the late 1800's. In the early part of the 20th century, however, the power of doctors practicing allopathic medicine (preferring drugs or surgery over natural remedies) grew through their participation in the Doctors Union, now known as the American Medical Association. The organization took over medical schools, the accreditation of physicians and influenced regulatory agencies as well as the mass media, countering the success of homeopaths. As a result, our generation has not heard of homeopathic success.

Homeopathy, which uses all-natural, non-toxic therapy designed to boost our bodies' own healing properties, is contrary to orthodox treatments that use toxic, non-natural treatments. The best of it incorporates the scientific method and the art of healing. A link to a video that briefly (4 minutes) discusses this history can be found here: http://www.youtube.com/watch?v=FPUqsZx5ARg&feature=player_embedded

Because the allopathic practices still dictate our medicine today, the natural, non-toxic forms of cancer treatment (such as the Gerson Therapy, Dr. Keller's Diet, Budwig Diet, Gonzalez/Isaacs protocol, etc.) are not leveraged in mainstream medicine. However, homeopathy was founded by a physician and is more in line with Hippocrates than what most of Western doctors today are practicing.

It has only been in this century that we have walked away from treating the whole person, to today's practice: one specialist to the next, treating each issue separately, instead of treating the totality of the individual.

This was an Aha! Moment.

THE FLEXNER REPORT

It is interesting to look at the link between a report that was commissioned in 1910 with what is going on in medicine today. The Flexner report precipitated the closing of medical schools that offered courses in homeopathy and natural medicine.

Abraham Flexner, a school teacher, was hired to research and prepare a report that would recommend the standard of care for medical schools – aligning medical education under a set of norms that emphasized laboratory research and the patenting of medicine. It was commissioned and funded by some of the most powerful drug and oil business partners in the industry: Rockefeller, Andrew Carnegie, J.P. Morgan and others.

The report of the Commission concluded that there were too many doctors and medical schools in America and recommended reducing the number of schools. The public outcry generated by the report convinced congress "to declare the AMA the only body with the right to grant medical school licenses in the United States." (Campaignforrealhealth.com) In all, more than 50% of schools closed.

While the report helped open eyes to needed improvements for hands-on learning, it also favored a strong bias of empirical science driven by pharmaceutical drugs, instead of taking into account whole-patient care or natural treatment options. The schools that taught holistic therapies were shut down.

That began the snowball effect that has brought us to where we are today: Individuals going from one specialist to the next, treating each issue separately, instead of treating the totality of the individual. An allegory (Town of Allopath) and most impactful story about allopathic medicine and its impact on a small town can be found at: http://www.naturalnews.com/008674.html. The animated parody of the Town of Allopath can be seen here: https://www.youtube.com/watch?v=97N18BTyj4w.

TESTIMONIAL

CHRIS WARK | Stage 3 Colon Cancer

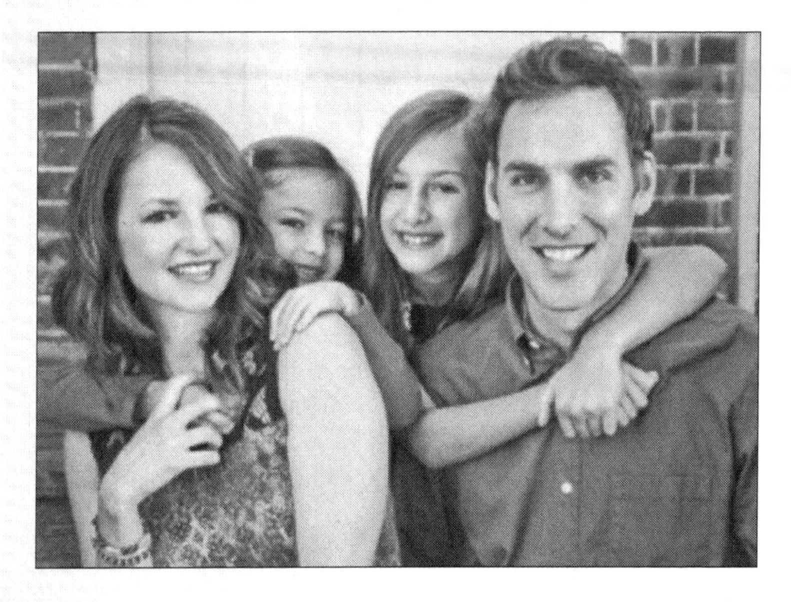

In 2003, I was a 26 year old newlywed, budding real estate entrepreneur, and part-time musician. Life was good. The last thing I expected was getting diagnosed with colon cancer!! But it happened. I was in shock! How could this be? This was not in my life plan! They said

I needed surgery to remove a golf ball size tumor, but likely would not need chemo. However, after surgery they said it was worse than they thought, stage 3, and I would need 9-12 months of chemo. What???? While in the hospital soon after surgery, I remember the first alarm that went off in my head. They gave me a sloppy joe for my first meal. Really? You took out 1/3 of my large intestine, yet mystery meat on a bun sounds like a good idea? The next flinch was when I asked the doctor what my diet should be when I went home. His advice to me was I could eat whatever I wanted, just don't lift anything heavier than a beer!

My wife and I have a strong faith in God and believe in the power of prayer. I was not comfortable at all with putting chemo in my body, so we prayed for guidance. Miraculously, the next day a book was on my front step from a man I had never met who lived in Alaska. God's Way to Ultimate Health by George Malkmus was the first book I read that opened my eyes to the cancer industry, nutritional therapy, juicing, and the raw vegan diet.

Faith is Choosing to Believe

I started right away on the raw diet. At this point, I told my wife I was not going to do chemo. It didn't take long for the phone to start ringing. Well intentioned family members were very concerned that I was not going to do conventional treatment. They actually did convince me to at least get an appointment with the oncologist just to see what he had to say. At the appointment, the doctor did most of the talking and I listened. He told me I had a 60% chance of making it 5 years if I took chemo. That sounded crazy to me! I asked him about the raw diet and he said I couldn't do that because it would fight the chemo! He also told me if I didn't get chemo I was insane! I asked him if there were any alternative therapies. He got very arrogant and said 'look I'm not saying all this because I need your business.' Business?????? After the picture he painted for me, and the fear he instilled, I was so upset I actually made an appointment to have a port put in to prepare for the chemo. I had walked in a confident man and walked out terrified.

After leaving the doctor's office in a state of terror, feeling confused and desperate for answers, my wife and I got in the car held hands, cried and once again prayed. I choked out a prayer for God to show us the path to follow. As the appointment date for the port got closer I started getting more and more apprehensive.

I finally told my wife I was not getting chemo, I knew there was a better way. From that point on I took on a lifestyle of overdosing on nutrients! I ate an organic/vegan diet. I juiced 64 oz a day of carrot/celery juice, made giant salads full of tons of vegetables, drank nutrient rich smoothies, and ate every organic fruit and vegetable I could get my hands on. My regime also included various exercise including a rebounder, stress management exercises and some supplements.

I have learned so much since then. FEAR is your enemy, do not be afraid! Cancer is actually a natural, normal process. The lump, bump, or lesion is a symptom. You aren't sick because you have cancer, you have cancer because you are sick! Many factors go into making us sick. The typical western diet of processed foods full of sugar, sodium, GMOs and unpronounceable ingredients are making us toxic and ill. We are overfed and malnourished. Stress is also a huge factor in making us sick. Another VERY IMPORTANT component to healing is to understand that in order for the body to heal physically we must also heal emotionally. Harboring emotions such as un-forgiveness, jealousy, resentment, bitterness, etc. is detrimental to our health. These are all immune suppressants that prohibit our bodies from achieving optimal wellness. God designed our miraculous bodies to heal themselves; we need to give them the tools to do so!

It has been 13 years since my wake-up call! I am cancer-free and have never been healthier! It's important to have a support system during this time. Healing Strong™ groups are a wonderful thing to be a part of! The power of the HealingStrong™ group comes from fostering a vibrant, synergistic, loving community where patients get inspiration and motivation, and are empowered with information to take action (or change direction), are encouraged to be strong, courageous and never give up.

Editor's Note:
Chris Wark has a very popular blog: **www.chrisbeatcancer.com**, is an international speaker, and creator of the healing cancer coaching program (Square One) that has helped thousands of people around the world on their own journey to heal strong and stay strong. In this program, Chris includes details on his successful journey with nutrition, supplements, detoxification and spiritual healing. It is one of the most powerful tools available for anyone facing a cancer diagnosis and want information on holistic strategies. Chris is a true champion, and a strong advocate for patients. He has impacted thousands and thousands of people's lives with his story and shared wisdom.

To access Chris Wark's Square One Modules:
https://sn188.infusionsoft.com/go/go/HealingStrong

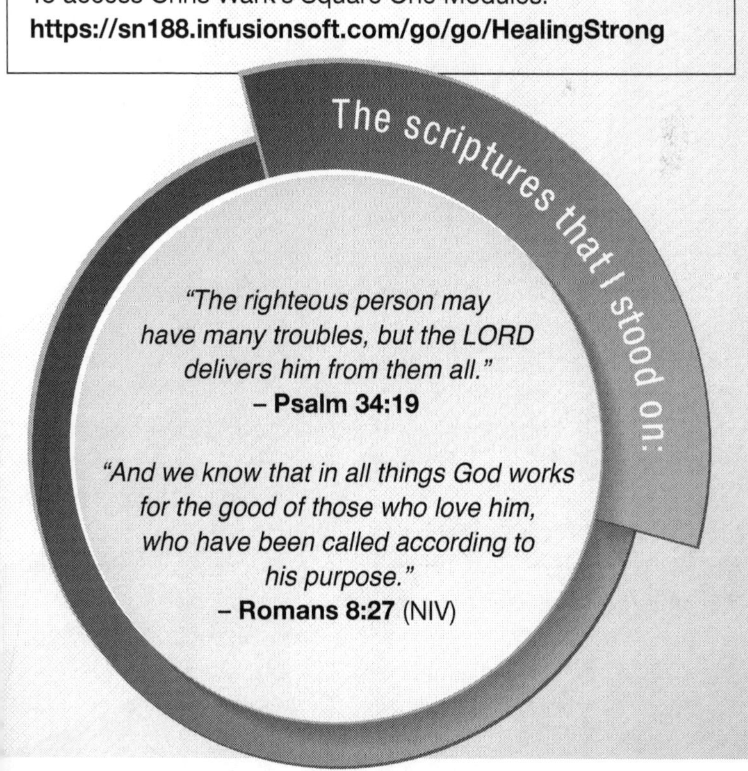

TESTIMONIAL

SARAH ANN COOPER

Pancreatic Cancer
Stage 4
HealingStrong™
Group Leader
Ormond Beach, FL

Write your sorrows in sand, and your blessings in stone.

– author unknown

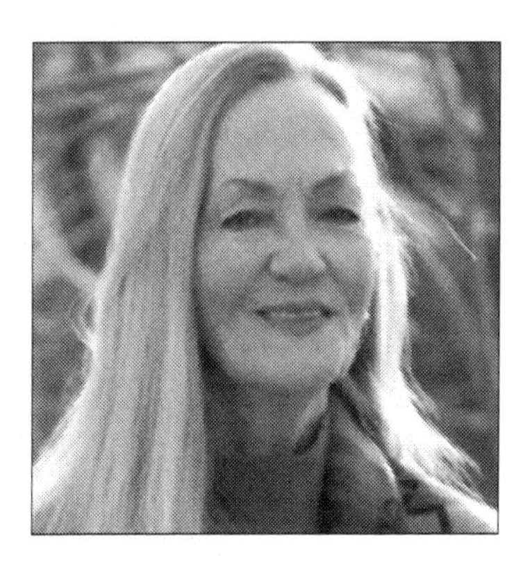

On December 5, 2000, a tumor mass of 3.2 cm was found in my pancreas by accident during a cat scan of my lungs and colon. I didn't even know where my pancreas was located. I was surprised and shocked especially since this was all as a result of a routine check-up. After meeting with two surgeons at Kaiser Permanente, I realized that I was facing a life threatening disease. They immediately wanted me to have surgery (called a Whipple). If I survived surgery then of course, chemo and radiation would follow. The best any Pancreatic Cancer patient could hope for was to extend their life 15 to 18 months. Without surgery, the life expectancy was 3 to 6 months. I considered the extent of the operation and the organs involved and I put off the surgery and started reading everything I could find from the AMA, the NCI and books by MD's and alternative medicine doctors. At that time, there was limited material to research as most doctors really feared getting involved in anything not approved by the AMA. However, I found enough to start a vitamin and herbal regimen.

I was determined to not have the surgery so I read and investigated everything on cancer and my cancer in particular. Needless to say, I asked for prayer from family and church leaders, attended healing conferences and listened for guidance from the Holy Spirit. My Kaiser doctor had all kinds of tests done in the hopes it was an endocrine tumor and not a carcinoma.

In February 2001 since I still refused surgery and chemo, my general practitioner, urged me to have a biopsy. Pathology at Kaiser and Mayo Clinic confirmed the mass as a carcinoma in the head of my pancreas or pancreatic cancer. While talking to a doctor in CA about a Rife machine, he directed me to a trial test being conducted by Dr. Gonzalez and Dr. Isaacs for alternative medicine and Columbia University Hospital for standard medicine.

I submitted all the blood test, cat scans and medical documentation to Columbia and was admitted to the trial, I thought. I flew to NY just to learn that I was not eligible for the trial program since I could have surgery even though I chose not to. Dr. Linda Isaacs and Dr. Nicholas Gonzalez showed compassion and offered me their services if I could just pay for the pills and other items I would need to follow the protocol. I jumped at the chance and have never looked back. I know in my spirit if I had chosen another route, I would not have lived to see my only granddaughter, Sarah, named after 5 generations of Sarah's, born and now 14 years old.

By this time my family had vacillated between wondering if I was in denial or just not understanding my choices. They were worried however they were standing with me on my decisions. Each of my children decided they would go with me on a trip to celebrate life. My husband, Jim, and I went to Mexico to a beautiful and peaceful resort for two weeks. My eldest daughter and her son enjoyed Disney World for a week with me. My son and I took a road trip from Denver to the coast of California from southern CA to the state line of Oregon and back by a different route. I had my protocol with me and kept faithfully on the regimen. Then my youngest daughter, her two sons and I traveled to Santa Fe and on to Taos NM. The trips, the sites and the love we shared were just wonderful beyond belief. There was no time to worry or fret. Only time to enjoy life and see the beautiful country God had given to us. Love of God, Love of family and Love of country and the beauty of it gave me the hope and faith to trust and listen to that quiet, still voice to keep going.

It has been 16 years since I was given my fatal news. I know people will say I'm crazy but the experience, the lessons I've learned, the people I've met and the walk with God is something I count as a blessing. If I could wash it all away, I would not. It's not all been easy however whose life is perfect. I've been in good health and able to do anything I wished to do including speaking to groups, teaching classes to others about alternative medicine, giving cancer patients hope and start writing a book.

Ann wrote the forward to Dr. Nicholas Gonzalez' book: *What Went Wrong: The Truth Behind the Clinical Trial of the Enzyme Treatment of Cancer.*

Recommended Resources:

The Complete Book of BIBLE PROMISES
by J. Stephen Lang

Knockout
by Suzanne Somers

What Went Wrong
by Nicholas J. Gonzalez, MD

One Man Alone
by Nicholas J. Gonzalez, MD

Cancer: Curing the Incurable, Without Surgery, Chemotherapy, or Radiation
by William Donald Kelley, DDS, MS

Editor's Note:
See Also Ann's Story and video interview at:
http://cancercompassalternateroute.com/testimonials/pancreatic-cancer-healed-with-natural-therapies

To locate Ann group in Ormond Beach, FL, or others like hers – go to the map and find the location you are interested at: **www.healingstrong.org/groups**

Aha! Moment #2 Current Cancer Treatments Aren't Working Well

SUZY'S PERSONAL PERSPECTIVE

Many people in my own family had lung cancer and the course of treatment was awful. My mother's last two and a half years were grueling and the radiation and chemotherapy she endured, I believe, killed her.

The last ten years of her life was wrought with peripheral neuropathy and cardiac failure due to the chemo drugs she took when initially diagnosed with stage 4 ovarian cancer.

The doctors treated her with the harshest of chemotherapy drugs, and several years later, evidence showed that the hospital had mixed up my mother's chart and cell slides with another woman on the same floor.

Unfortunately, the drugs had already done the damage. My mother could not walk without a cane, and spent unending sleepless nights from the pain of the neuropathy caused from the chemotherapy drugs. I believe the lung cancer that showed up later in her life was due to the chemotherapy, and oncologists today will agree.

Before I went any further with my treatment, I wanted to know what conventional medicine was doing for cancer, and whether it was really making a difference. I thought about my own family. Before me, twelve family members were diagnosed with cancer. Of those, ten died of the disease. I was number 13 in my family and the odds were stacked against me. Really digging into the data and research led me to Aha! Moment #2.

Considering all the advances in technology, research, surgical procedures, and pharmaceuticals, the cancer outcome data is startling.

- Within the past 50 years, there has only been a 5% drop in the death rate in cancer patients. (Jemal, A. et al. CA Cancer J Clin, 2010) However, the incidence of cancer is growing at an alarming rate. In 1975, one out of seven people would be diagnosed with cancer. Today the cancer rate is one out of two for men and the cancer rate is fast approaching the same ratio for women. In 2010, the report for the President's Cancer Panel, a three-person panel that reports to the U.S. president on the National Cancer Program, said approximately 41 percent of Americans will be diagnosed with cancer during their lifetime Look at the incidence rates vs. mortality rates (death rates since 1975). This is alarming.

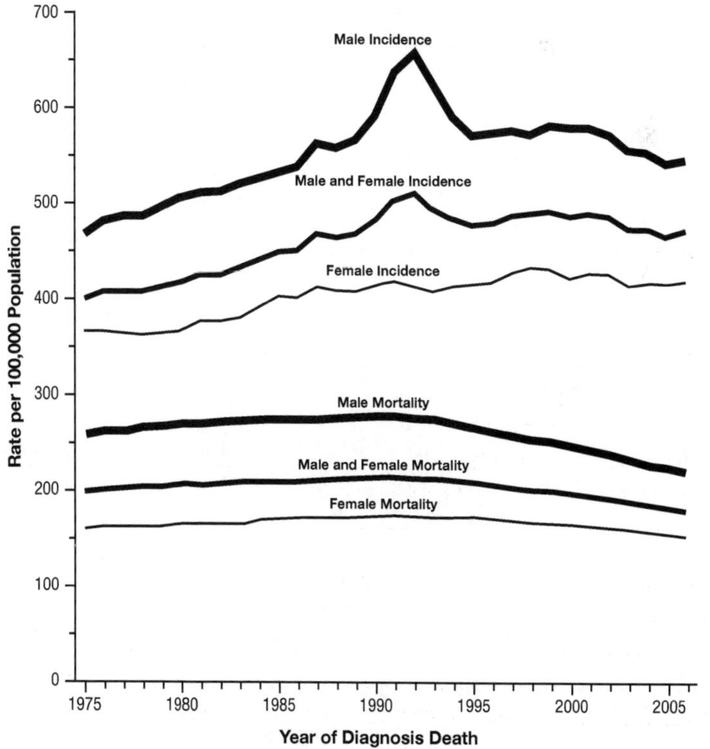

- According to the World Health Organization, cancer is a leading cause of death worldwide and it is the second most common cause of death in the United States. It accounted for 7.4 million deaths (around 13% of all deaths) in 2004 (statistics published in 2009). Deaths from cancer worldwide are projected to continue rising, with an estimated 12 million deaths in 2030.
- Data from the National Center for Health Statistics show that death rates over the past 60 years — the number of deaths adjusted for the age and size of the population — plummeted for heart disease, stroke, and influenza and pneumonia. But for cancer, they barely budged. (NY Times, April 2009)
- A separate report in the New England Journal of Medicine, published in 1986, assessed progress against cancer in the United States during the years 1950-1982. Despite progress against some rare forms of cancer, which account for one to two percent of total deaths caused by the disease, the report found that the overall death rate had increased substantially since 1950. "The main conclusion we draw is that some 35 years of intense effort focused largely on improving treatment must be judged a qualified failure," the report concluded. "We are losing the war against cancer."
- Chemotherapy has a mere 2.3% success rate at healing cancers in America. This is according to a study based out of Sydney, Australia, conducted by the Australian Medical Association. The authors found that the contribution of chemotherapy to 5-year survival in adults was 2.3 percent in Australia, and 2.1 percent in the USA. They emphasize that, for reasons explained in detail in the study, these figures "should be regarded as the upper limit of effectiveness". This was an important paper, published in the December 2004 issue of Clinical Oncology. (https://www.ncbi.nlm.nih.gov/pubmed/15630849).
- Ralph Moss, in a 1995 interview, emphasized that chemotherapy is effective in only 2 to 4% of cancers – Hodgkin's disease, Acute Lymphocytic Leukemia (ALL, childhood leukemia), Testicular cancer, and Choriocarcinoma. (http://www.livelinks.com/sumeria/canc/rmoss.html)
- There is no scientific evidence for chemotherapy being able to extend in any appreciable way the lives of patients suffering from the most common organic cancers, which accounts for 80% of all cancers. (Dr Ulrich Abel. 1990)

- In the book *The Topic of Cancer: When the Killing Has to Stop*, Dick Richards cites autopsy studies that show cancer patients died from cancer treatments before the tumors themselves had a chance to kill them.

Even more startling to me than the statistics showing that the incidence of cancer is growing, and modern treatments are not proving much more effective than they were decades ago, was discovering the relationship physicians have with allopathic treatments such as chemotherapy.

- Since 1971, $2 TRILLION has been spent on conventional cancer research and treatments. Interestingly, I read a study where **most (75%) of the oncologists who were surveyed by the McGill Cancer Center scientists would not take the chemo that they recommend to their patients lung cancer patients if they were also diagnosed with lung cancer**. *W J Mackillop, G K Ward & B O'Sullivan, "The use of expert surrogates to evaluate clinical trials in non-small cell lung cancer," British Journal Cancer 1986; 54:661-667*
- Chemotherapeutic drugs are **the only classification of drugs** that the doctor who prescribes the protocol for the patient actually gets a direct cut. How is that? The doctor buys it from the pharmaceutical company and sells it back to the patient – at whatever profit he or she wants.

While it is important to note that accurate data analysis depends greatly on looking at how the data is presented (if you ask someone from HealingStrong™ about this, we can walk you through this), there is no doubt that not much has changed in this century to improve cancer prevention or cancer mortality. **This knowledge, coupled with my own personal family experience of only a 17% survival rate from conventional cancer treatments, was definitely an Aha! Moment for me!**

TESTIMONIAL

BAILEY O'BRIEN

Melanoma
Stage 4

"If you're going through hell, keep going."

– Winston Churchill

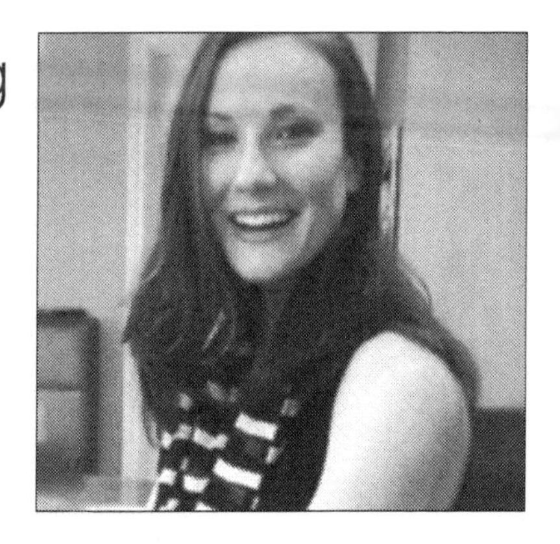

My journey began when I was 17 and in my first semester of college. After discovering a suspicious mole, I found out I had malignant melanoma that had spread to a lymph node. My first steps were to undergo conventional treatments, including surgery and interferon to help prevent the cancer from returning. However, these conventional means failed and it came back at the beginning of my senior year.

For the second time, I went through conventional treatments, this time surgery and radiation. Just two weeks after finishing radiation I felt a little bump under my chin. A biopsy confirmed that it was my melanoma, back again. I was devastated and frustrated that after all I had been through – my treatments and surgeries, losing half of my ear and missing out on my best year as a student-athlete – it had all been for nothing; I was back at square one. My doctor ordered a scan that confirmed the tumor under my chin as well as six other tumors in my neck, lung, and spine, now at stage 4. And when I found out that I didn't qualify for the most promising drug, with very little promise for a future,

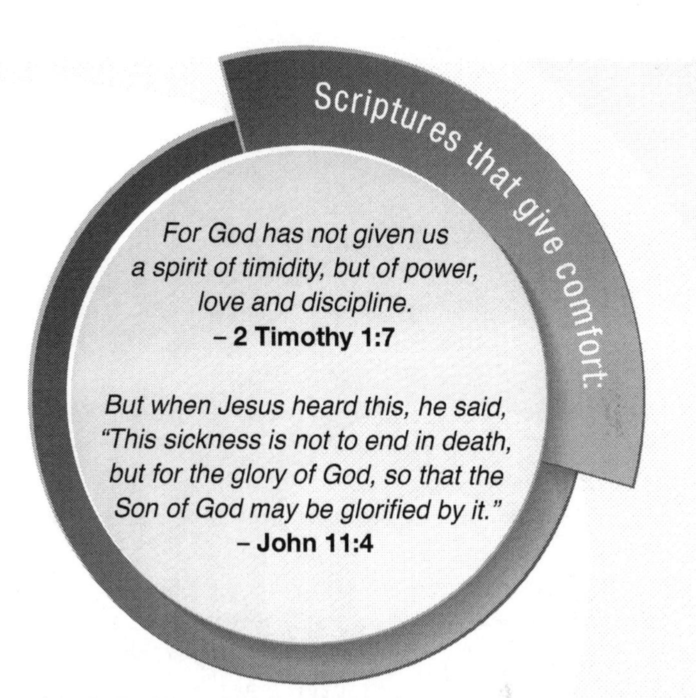

I thought of all of the doctors who were out there and how none of them offered the hope I was looking for.

I remember being in my dorm room and looking outside of my beautiful window onto the Boston skyline. I was desperate for a new angle and my mom told me of her friend that was an advocate for natural and alternative treatments. She truly believed that I could be cured, and I was ready to hear what she had to say.

After consulting with many different doctors and doing one last brief round of Temodar, a chemo pill, my mom and I decided that my best shot for natural treatment was a hospital in Mexico. My treatments would include an eighteen month commitment to a modified Gerson Therapy; this included juices, a plant-based diet, and detoxification using coffee enemas. I would also be introduced to Coley fluid, an autologous vaccine, high dose vitamin C, Laetrile (B17), liver shots, and supplements. With this treatment I was given a greater than 60% chance of success.

Terrified of the unknown but resolved, my mom and I left for a three week stay in Mexico. The doctors and staff were warm and friendly and we felt safe in their care. The diet and treatments were difficult but bearable, and by the time I left the lump under my chin had vanished. I continued my treatments and diet at home, and after another 3 weeks had a scan. It showed no signs of cancer. After praying to a God that I didn't know at the time, I was healed.

Today, I know that God showed me what I needed to do, and by His amazing grace, I was healed!

Some resources that I have found to be of value over the years include:

- The Gerson Research Organization (Gar and Christeene Hildenbrand; gerson-research.org)
- PubMed and PMC (https://www.ncbi.nlm.nih.gov/)
- *A Cancer Therapy: Results of 50 Cases* by Dr. Max Gerson
- *Radical Remission* by Dr. Kelly Turner (radicalremission.com)
- *One Man Alone: An Investigation of Nutrition, Cancer, and William Donald Kelley* by Dr. Nicholas Gonzalez
- *Nutrition and the Autonomic Nervous System: The Scientific Foundations of the Gonzalez Protocol* by Dr. Nicholas Gonzalez

---

For a video interview of Bailey sharing her story, please go to:
https://www.youtube.com/watch?v=6tRhkYQ9q-g

Bailey O'Brien now shares her journey and experience as a Certified Integrative Nutrition Health Coach, helping others through their own journeys to heal and stay strong.
www.baileyobrien.com

TESTIMONIAL

TIAH TOMLIN

Triple Negative Breast Cancer HealingStrong™ Group Leader Atlanta, GA

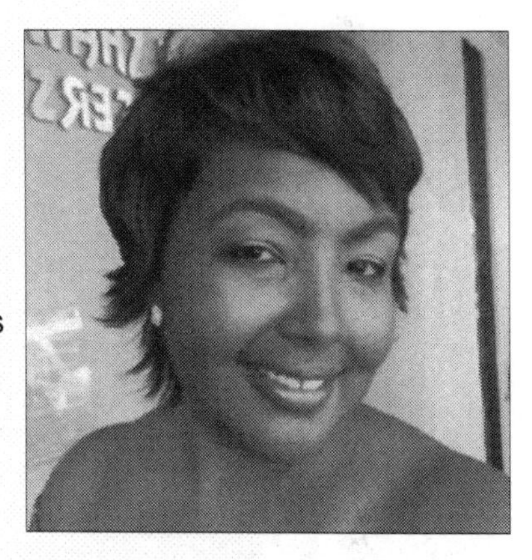

Editor's Note:
Tiah is an active mentor, group leader, and Advisory Board Member for HealingStrong™. Her story of healing through an integrative approach represents so many participants at our HealingStrong™ meetings. Today, she actively encourages people through her many activities to examine closely the daily habits that lead to disease and poor health outcomes, and how each can regain their health and wellness moving forward.

Cancer startled me on a normal workday. I rushed home from the gym to jump in the shower and get ready to attend an event. I was very good about doing breast self-exams regularly in the shower, and just expected to feel the same thing that I felt just a week ago - nothing. But something was different. Quickly moving my fingers across my breast, I felt something hard and my heart sank.

A few days later, after several tests, my doctor called me. As she began to talk, all I heard was carcinoma. I broke. Just days before this, my business partner and I had just announced our company, My Style Matters, partnership with the Veterans Empowerment Organization and the American Cancer Society to raise awareness for Prostate cancer and collect suits for veterans via our fun run event called the "5K Suit Run™." We had work to do for others battling this disease. I was in shock. All I could think of was "Why me? Why now? Why my family? How am I going to tell my family? What about the My Styles Matters team and the 5K Suit Run? This can't be happening. What about my job: I can't afford to lose it! Where did I miss the mark?

She must have sensed my lost feeling because she said we could discuss it the next day. I hung up the phone and cried. As I wept, I could hear God telling me "You can either sit there and wallow in your grief or you can get up and fight. Now, get up!" God has always been there for my family. My father had a major stroke in 2011 and had a miraculous recovery. My brother was diagnosed with stage 4 testicular cancer at 32, also in 2011, and is still living and is cancer free, despite having been given only six months to live. I hoped God would do the same for me. Sobbing, I began to speak to my spirit..."Get up! Get up!" I went from crying and hurting to praising and worshiping... "Yet will I trust You Lord! Yet will I trust You!"

We met with the Cancer Care team within a few days of receiving that dreadful call. There we learned that the cancer was aggressive and that I would have to undergo 8 rounds chemotherapy, have a lumpectomy or mastectomy and possibly 33 rounds of radiation. They also informed us about the nasty side effects that I could experience. Hearing this, coupled with my background in chemistry, it was then I knew that I did not want to undergo chemotherapy. I reached out to a naturopath to help guide me. When he told how much it would cost, I knew I could not afford completely going the alternative route. My family and I prayed about it and committed to just stand on faith no matter what I felt, saw or heard. I believed that God had the final say over my life. I told myself to remain positive at all times, finding ways to laugh through the journey because the "Joy of the Lord was and is my Strength!"

Two weeks before I started chemo, I researched as much as I could and joined every alternative/holistic Facebook group I could find. I knew that I needed to make lifestyle changes immediately to fight this disease. Therefore, I got rid of all of my household and personal care products. The next step I took was purchasing a Vitamix blender and an Omega juicer. Once chemotherapy treatment started, each week my fierce fighting team would fast and my father would send out a prayer and encouraging word to help us get started. I began eating salads, steamed spinach, kale and fruits. I drank keifer, homemade juices, alkaline water and every so often, a 2 oz. shot of wheatgrass. When I finally finished chemotherapy in October, I retained this diet. The following month, I had a lumpectomy with the removal of two lymph nodes. My pathology results came back negative and I was cancer-free. But being that I was diagnosed with Triple negative breast cancer and had a lumpectomy, the doctor prescribed 33 rounds of radiation.

Once it was all over, I knew that I needed to continue to rebuild my body. I stopped taking all of my pain medication and replaced it with essential oils and began taking vitamins and supplements such as B17, CDB Oil, and Frankincense. I also purchased an IR-sauna and sat in it several times a day followed by a detox bath. I began to walk one mile at a time and worked my way up to five. I also incorporated coffee enemas, rebounding, and lymphatic brushing into my healing regimen. As for diet, I decided to attend a 10-day raw food program and since attending, I have been able to incorporate a few things into my rebuilding process. I truly believe that these lifestyle changes are necessary to help heal our bodies. Six months after I finished all of my treatments, I began notice that my test results were backsliding. So I took the next few months and made more drastic changes; just to test out the theory that a holistic approach really works. When I went back for my three month checkup, all of my results looked great. In that very moment, I knew that this is the life I need to live. Currently, I am working on making changes in my diet altogether for the long haul, eliminating meat.

Since the diagnosis, I've been busy helping others fight. I started a Facebook group called My Breast Years Ahead - Atlanta, helping women affected by any type of cancer in the Atlanta area connect and support one another. In 2016, I participated in the Cancer Moonshot Summit and became one of the team advisory members and chapter leaders for HealingStrong™. I also joined the Check It Out! Program to help educate young high school girls about breast health. I was chosen to be a Young Program Advocate for Living Beyond Breast Cancer as well as co-facilitator of Sisters By Choice – 40 & Under Support group. In addition, I started the Kick Can't-cer Care Kit project where my company, My Style Matters, has partnered with I Will Survive, Inc, to help educate newly diagnosed survivors about making lifestyle changes and providing them with the tools to do so by providing a care kit containing non-toxic household and personal care items along with non-GMO and organic snacks and beverages. Recently, I received the Charge Up Award from Charge Up Campaign for my dedication to being a beacon of HOPE as well as fighting against what I call 'Can't-cer' by speaking out about prevention and increasing awareness around making lifestyle changes.

Proverbs 3:5-6 (NIV)

"Trust in the LORD with all your heart and lean not on your own understanding; in all your ways submit to him, and he will make your paths straight."

TESTIMONIAL

KAY HAHN | Stage 4 Pancreatic Cancer

I constantly repeated verses stating that my faith had healed me and for me to believe and not doubt.

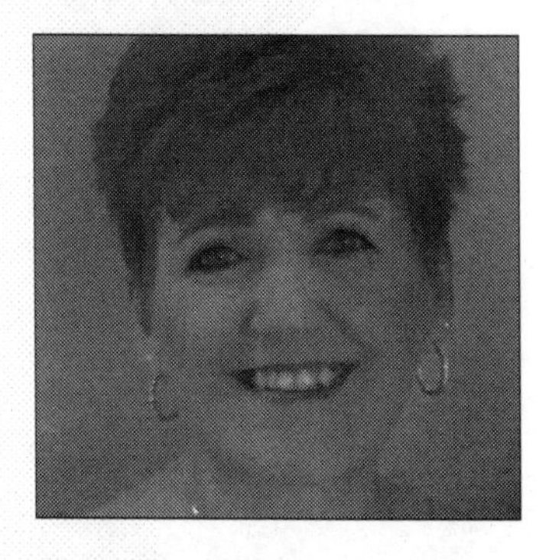

In January, 2012, I was diagnosed with pancreatic cancer, metastasized to the liver, a total of 9 tumors that they could see. The diagnosing doctor told me I should get my affairs in order. My immediate thought was Patrick Swayze only lived a few months after being diagnosed… I won't be here by March. But I knew someone bigger than this doctor, someone bigger than this malfunction in my body. I told the doctor, "No, God's going to take care of it. I am going to be alright." Six years earlier I had a life threatening health issue but I trusted God for my healing. In addition I had seen the destructive nature of conventional treatment in my family and others, I knew there was no one else who was going to be able to do anything for me, besides God.

I didn't want to do chemo, I seriously did not believe I needed it. I right away began researching cures for cancer and I found Dr. Max Gerson and Nurse Rene Caisse. But my family was scared and were conditioned to listen to our doctor. So in the next ten months I went through seven kinds of chemo, three oncologists, and three hospitals, including MD Anderson. All it accomplished was to almost kill me on several occasions.

Through this whole time it kept going over in my mind, along with continual "God Winks", to keep my eyes on Jesus and to always Believe and speak and walk in that Belief. The mental fight is half the battle. Not every day was easy but I trusted Him that He provided everything we were going to need in this life in the garden.

In September 2012, I had a very old, very fanciful dressed woman come up to me and tell me I needed to go to the health food store on the other end of town. I didn't know this woman or that there even was a health food store in our town for over 30 years. But I still went and it changed my life. Even though I was in my last clinical trial, I started taking supplements to nourish my immune system. In December I opted to stop the chemo because at that point my body had been through every kind of awful side effect that was possible. I believe the chemo was destroying my body from the bone marrow outward to the point where it hurt to do simple things like stepping up on a curb. After all that treatment, my doctor told me there had been no improvement from a whole year of chemo. After everything I had been through, my body was in worse shape than when I started.

A few months later, a friend wrote me and told me about a friend of hers healing from cancer using the Gerson Therapy. My body was terribly broken from all the conventional treatment. I had been near death and didn't know what to think, but in her loving determination, she started sending me boxes of everything I needed, a juicer, supplements and even a coffee enema kit. In February, I started the Gerson Therapy. Two and a half weeks later I had a 20% decrease in tumors. Three months after that, there was more decrease. Six months after that, I was feeling great and my doctor said if I wasn't going to listen to conventional methods there was no point in me coming back. So I haven't been back since December 2013. I believe our bodies were made to heal and God provided all we need to nourish and heal our bodies.

I have tried other protocols because my tumor markers would go up and down and my HCG was staying steady. I didn't see a drastic drop in both of those tests until Aug. 2015 when I found the books, 80/10/10 and The Raw Cure. I began eating a raw, mostly fruit diet and my body started resetting itself. In about eight weeks my tests were all just above the normal mark, even my blood sugar. This made me realize of the all the helpful supplements I took, the good things God gave me from the earth, are the most important aspects in nourishing and healing my body. Along with trusting Him, Believing His word, the power of His sacrifice, and speaking the truth of His extravagant love for me was a critical part of my healing. This experience has changed me, I've learned how much God loves me and now I can honestly say I would not have wanted to go through the rest of my life without this experience.

I am so thankful I did not choose to go the way of destruction, instead I chose the way of nourishing life. I still thank Him daily for my healing.

Resources that were helpful for me included:

www.chrisbeatcancer.com
www.cancertutor.com
www.fullyraw.com

80/10/10 by Dr. Douglas Graham
The Raw Cure by Jesse Jacoby
Cancer: Step Outside of the Box by Ty Bollinger

Verse of encouragement:

"Do not be afraid... you will not have to fight this battle... take up your positions; stand firm and see the deliverance the Lord will give you... Give thanks to the Lord for his love endures forever... was at peace for his God had given him rest."

– 2 Chronicles 20:15-30

TESTIMONIAL

IVELISSE PAGE | Stage 4 Colon Cancer

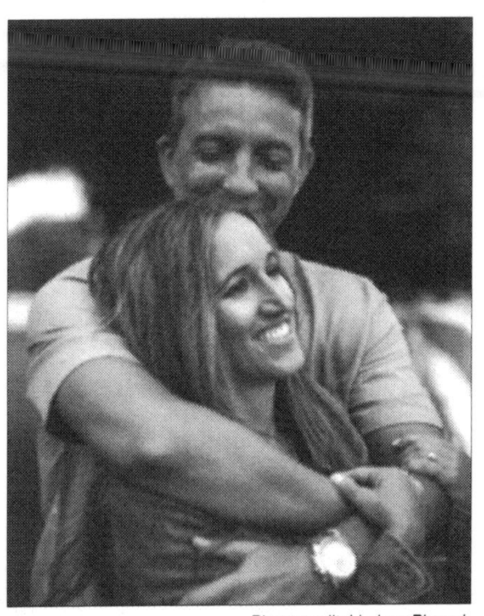

Photo credit: Lindsey Plevyak

In the fall of 2008 I was diagnosed with stage 4 colon cancer; I was the very same age and had the very same type of cancer that took my father's life, my grand-mother's life, and half of her siblings as well.

I was in complete shock as I thought I knew what to look for. I had been diligent of following my doctor's orders of getting a colonoscopy every 5 years and I did not experience a single symptom except extreme fatigue. This lead to the discovery that I was severely anemic and a simple blood test resulted in me being rushed to the hospital for a blood transfusion as my organs could have failed at any moment. Doctors were baffled and ran every test imaginable to figure out the cause. One physician even ruled out colon cancer because I had just had a colonoscopy 3 years prior. And yet it was a colonoscopy to "rule it out" that discovered the cancer. They also found that I had Lynch Syndrome, which only affects 3% of patients with colon cancer. This causes the cancer to grow and metastasize very rapidly, often becoming cancerous and dangerous in as little as two years versus the typical 10 years.

Tears began to flow, fear began to set in, and the thought of not seeing my four children grow up and growing old with my husband was overwhelming. I was overcome with emotion. Some people say that God won't give us anything we can't handle, but I believe that He often allows situations that are too much for us to handle – alone. It's in these times that we realize how much we need each other and most importantly, our need for God becomes obvious. And, we learn to trust and rely on the one who created us.

My dad's story kept ringing in my ears- diagnosed at 37, dead at 39. I had to convince myself that my dad's story was not my story; that my outcome could be different. But truthfully, a big part of me believed I was on the same path. I realized quickly that there was a choice to make. Would I give in to the fear or would I live by my faith and fight?

So in the days ahead I fought the fear that tried to grip me each day by filling my mind with His word. I decided to engage my faith and fight. I kept reminding myself of whom I was in Christ. I focused on the capability of my God instead of the challenge of cancer. I regularly read out-loud, often several times a day, the "I will have not fear" prayer that my husband, Jimmy, compiled for me. And the fear… it relented! I went back to what I knew. God did not give me a spirit of fear, but one of power, love and a sound mind. He promised me that He would never fail me or leave me. He promised to be faithful EVEN when I am all but out of faith. And, He told me to be strong and courageous, to quit being terrified or discouraged, and to trust in Him.

We also came to see the importance of having a team of doctors, both conventional and complementary, which would work together to heal the whole person. Discovering that the survivorship of stage 4 colon cancer with metastasis to the liver was less than 8%, Jimmy and I made the decision to forgo chemotherapy and radiation, as it would not have increased my chances of survival.

On the conventional side of my treatments, I had incredible surgeons who removed the cancer from my colon and liver, and I had an oncologist who monitored me with scans and blood work. Jimmy and I interviewed several oncologists, but we chose Dr. Diaz because he was willing to individualize my care, and humble enough to consider our complementary, holistic approach. And, truly believed I could get better!

On the complementary side, I changed my internal environment with the help of Dr. Hinderberger to fight any remaining cancer after surgeries with a high alkaline diet, homeopathy, cancer fighting supplements, and Mistletoe injections.

By God's grace these tools helped me win my battle with cancer and remain cancer-free today! After facing, fighting and overcoming cancer, I was compelled to reach out to patients facing similar challenges that I encountered in my fight against cancer.

Even though my husband had spent over 20 years in the health and wellness industry, we found it extremely difficult to find reliable resources to heal the whole person – physically, spiritually, mentally, and emotionally. Believe Big (BelieveBig.org) was established in 2011 to bridge the gap between conventional and complementary medicine for fighting cancer. Our focus is to educate individuals on a comprehensive approach to cancer prevention and treatment, connect patients with physicians trained in mistletoe therapy and the resources necessary to help them advocate for their own health, provide spiritual support to help patients overcome fear and anxiety, and overcome cancer with the Mistletoe Clinical trial in collaboration with Johns Hopkins University School of Medicine.

Some resources that I have found to be of value over the years include:

The Metabolic Approach to Cancer by Dr. Nasha

Radical Remission by Dr. Kelly Turner

50 Days of Hope by Lynn Eib

www.BelieveBig.org

www.RemissionNutrition.com

To read or print a copy of the I Will Have No Fear prayer, go to: **http://believebig.org/prayers**

For a video interview of Ivelisse sharing her story, go to: **https://www.youtube.com/watch?v=xsiFPKBgY3c**

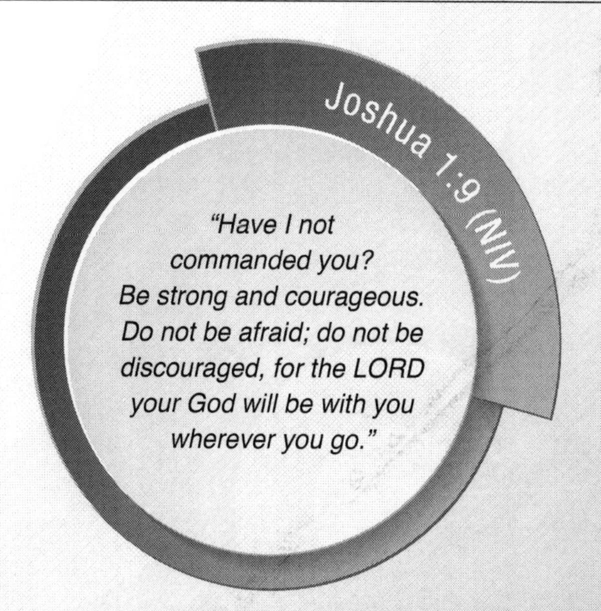

Aha! Moment #3 Cancer is a Process, Not a Thing!

It makes sense that in order to reverse the disease, we need to look at the primary problems and reverse those. Somewhere along the way, we have learned that cancer is the tumor, the affected lymph node, or the metastasis to the other organs.

My Aha! Moment came when I learned something a little different and quite surprising about cancer.

Cancer is a process, not a thing! Some of the best research that we have done on our cancer journey breaks down the cancer process as one of simplicity and something that made for an Aha! Moment.

Without going into the biological or metabolic explanations, I have provided some excerpts that helped shift my thinking and lead me to a healing strong journey that treated the systemic process, not the thing. Below are explanations of cancer, with the references, that made for a shift in my thinking and approach to treatment.

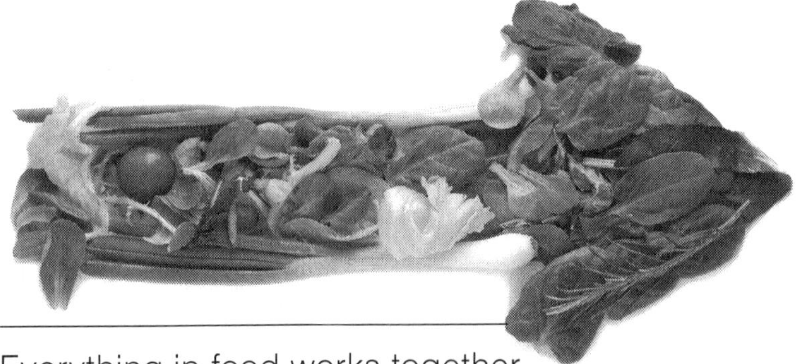

Everything in food works together, operating through a symphony of coordinated reactions to create health or disease.

EXAMPLE
1
Taken directly from
Cancer Ignorance by
Carol Morrison-Kelley, M.D., F.A.C.C.
William D. Kelley, D.D.S., M.S.)

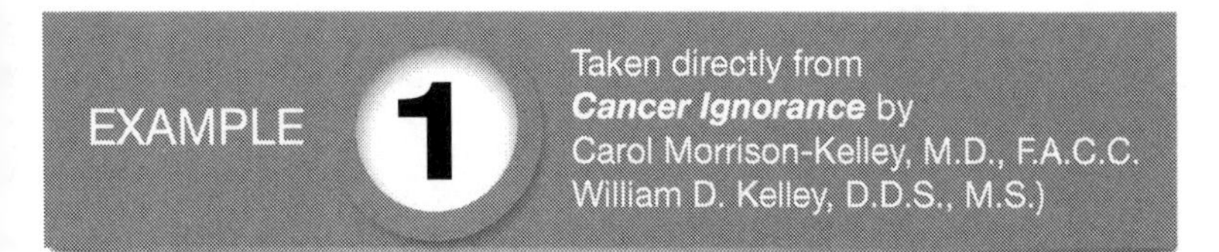

What Cancer is Not: Cancer is not those lumps and bumps that we have been so programmed to fear and freak out over if we find one on our body. Cancer is not a malignant tumor mass, which doctors, in their cancer ignorance, erroneously call cancer. This is one of the reasons we have so much "cancer". The physician does not know what cancer is. How could he properly treat it? The physicians, both orthodox and alternative, only know how to mistreat malignant tumor masses and blood and lymph abnormalities which is not even cancer.

What Cancer Is: "Cancer is a process - not an object. A diabetic going untreated will destroy his liver, kidneys, lungs, develop a gangrenous limb and go blind. The physician who performs a liver, lung and kidney transplant is not treating diabetes. The physician who amputates the gangrenous limb is not treating diabetes. The physician who prescribes a "seeing-eye dog" is not treating diabetes. The physician who describes insulin is not treating diabetes. The diabetic who gives himself insulin and changes his diet is properly treating his own diabetic condition.

The orthodox physician who uses surgery, radiation and chemotherapy is not treating cancer. The alternative "doctor" who prescribes herbs, shark cartilage, black salve, laetrile, vitamins, etc. is not treating cancer. The Chinese doctor who prescribes six cockroaches and three grasshoppers daily is not treating cancer. These items may help something else in one's body, but will not properly treat one's cancer.

Drs. Kelley and Kelley object of ***Metabolic Medicine's Cancer Cure Program*** is to supply the body with adequate pancreatin to properly digest food, stop this disease process, and rid the body of any and all malignant tumor cells. This is the proper, normal, physiological method of taking care of the disease process we correctly call cancer.

EXAMPLE
2
Taken Directly from
The China Study
by T. Colin Campbell, PhD

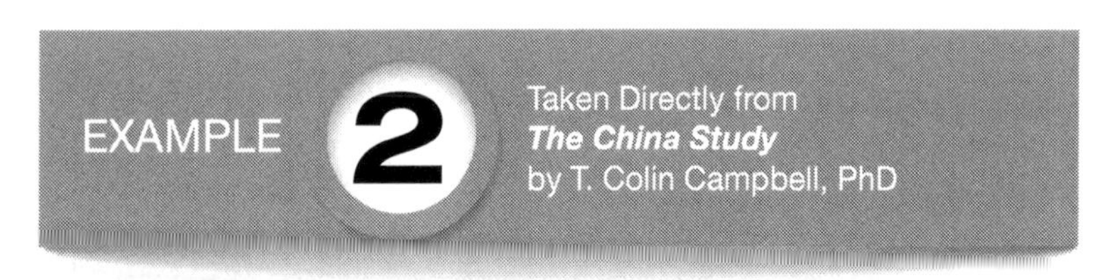

Everything in food works together to create health or disease. The important story here is how the effects of food – both good and bad – operate through a symphony of coordinated reactions to prevent diseases like prostate cancer. In discovering the existence of these networks, we sometimes wonder which specific function comes first and which comes next. We tend to think of these reactions within the network as independent. But this surely misses the point. What impresses me is the multitude of reactions working together in so many ways to produce the same effect: in this case, to prevent disease. There is no single "mechanism" that fully explains what causes diseases such as cancer. Indeed, it would be foolish to even think along these lines.

Food as key to health represents a powerful challenge to conventional medicine, which is fundamentally built on drugs and surgery. The widespread communities of nutrition professionals, researchers and doctors are, as a whole, either unaware of this evidence or reluctant to share it. Because of these failings, Americans are being cheated out of information that could save their lives.

EXAMPLE
3
Taken Directly from
Cancer Step Outside the Box
by Ty Bollinger

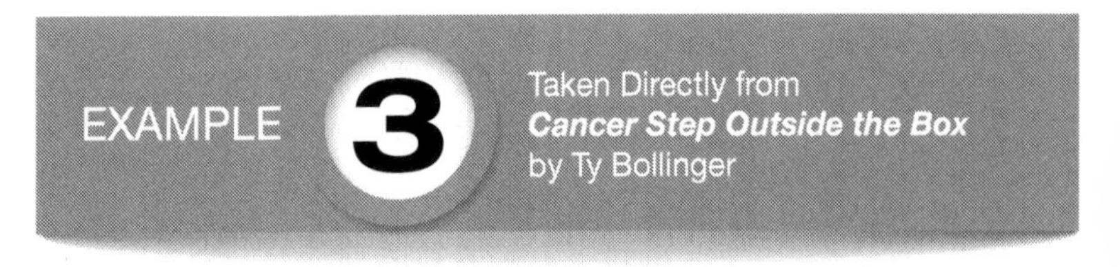

Ty Bollinger's book provides many illustrations of cancer in layman's terms that helps one to understand the "totality" of the disease and the absurdity of treating the tumor only. One of my favorites is his description of the "tumor tizzy." It is an oversimplification of the cancer process, but it certainly helped contribute to this Aha! Moment:

The Cancer Industry is in a "tumor tizzy." Most practitioners are so obsessed with shrinking the size of a tumor that they miss the mark completely. You see, chemotherapy does shrink tumors; that is true. However, despite the fact that oncologists are successfully able to shrink tumors, oftentimes the cancer patient still dies. But why? The reason is the tumor size has nothing to do with curing cancer. The tumor is like the "check engine" light in your car. It appears only after a problem has developed, but the light itself is not the problem. Do you smash the light, or do you attempt to fix the underlying problem? A tumor is just a signal that something has gone terribly wrong in the body… it is just the tip of the iceberg.

EXAMPLE
4
Taken Directly from
Healing the Gerson Way
by Charlotte Gerson

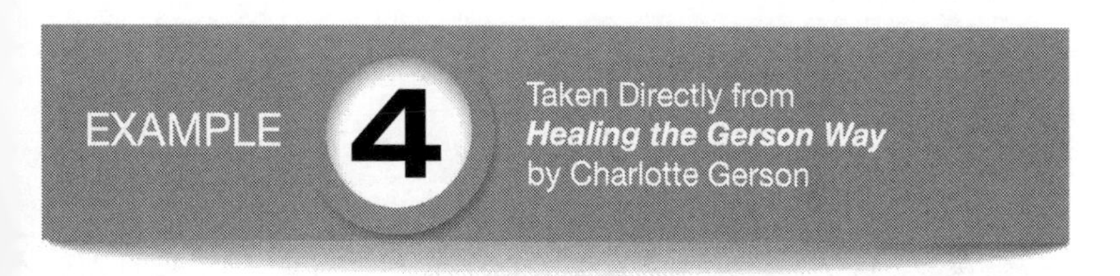

We must find our way back to an unadulterated natural lifestyle and learn how to restore our health by dealing with the causes, not just the symptoms, of our problems. The basic principle of the Gerson way of healing is totality. It means taking into account the entire organism and dealing with all its problems and weaknesses, not honing in on just one symptom or organ, as if it were independent from the rest of the body.

The body has a system of defenses that maintain homeostasis, the state of dynamic equilibrium of the internal environment. It is the disturbance of this equilibrium that starts the process of cell deterioration, and the disturbance itself can be caused by various chemicals, etc.

Cancer cannot occur in a normally functioning body because its defenses recognize and destroy any malignant cell that may develop or do not allow it to come into being at all. The immune system plays the leading role in the group of defenses. It recognizes a malignant cell as a foreign invader and attacks and destroys it, as it would any intruding germ or virus. However, the immune system, along with the other defenses (eg. enzyme and hormone systems and the proper mineral balances), consists of organs and glands that need proper nutrients, which can function only if they are not blocked by toxins. When those conditions don't apply, the defenses are unable to fulfill their task, and there is nothing to stop the malignant cell from surviving and multiplying.

Therefore, most importantly, the disappearance of the tumor only means that the responses have been restored to the point of re-

---

The immune system plays the leading role in the group of defenses. It recognizes malignant cell as a foreign invader and attacks and destroys it.

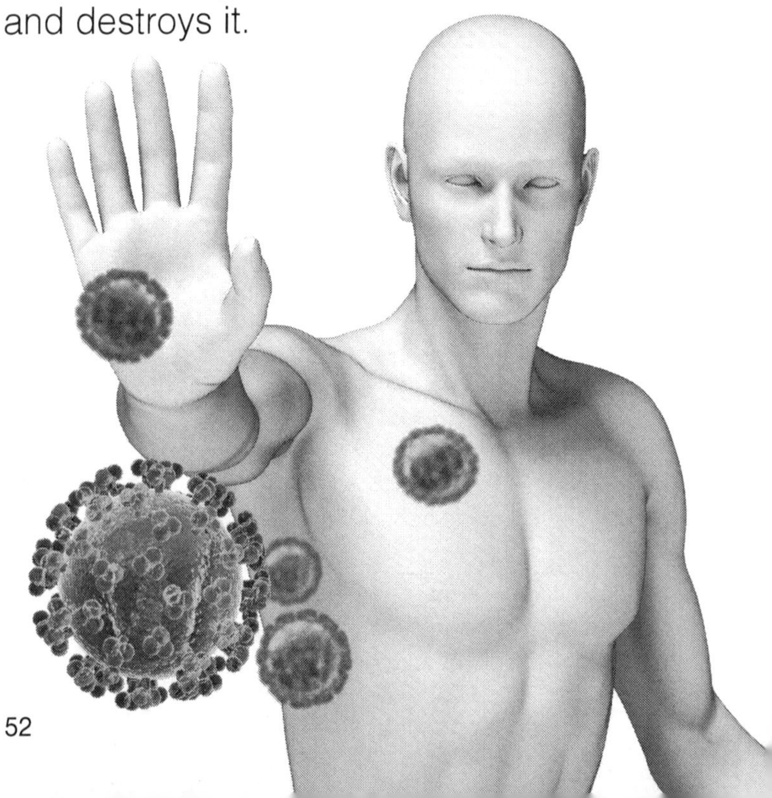

moving the threat to the patient's life, but that does not equal healing. Total healing can only occur when all the patient's organs have been restored, literally rebuilt, with the best organic foods and continued detoxification. Healing is only complete when the damaged toxic liver is cleansed and rebuilt to as near normal as possible.

"The great advantage of knowing the prime cause of a disease is that it can then be attacked logically and over a broad front. This is particularly important in the case of cancer, with its numerous secondary and remote causes, and because it is often stated that in man alone there are over one hundred well-known and quite different kinds of cancer, usually with the implication that therefore we will have to find one or several hundred bases for prevention and treatment, and usually without any realization that this need not necessarily be the case now that we know that **all cancers studied have a characteristic metabolism in common, a prime cause**."

– **Dr. Otto Warburg**
Two Time Nobel Prize Winner

Understanding how cancer works as a process – not a thing – was critical in helping me understand why I needed to approach my cancer treatment holistically. Natural therapies were beginning to make a whole lot more sense to me. It was an Aha! Moment, for sure!

> The tumor is like the "check engine" light in your car. It appears only after a problem has developed, but the light itself is not the problem.

TESTIMONIAL

IVETTE VALENZUELA

Adenoid Cystic Carcinoma HealingStrong™ Group Leader Falls Church, VA

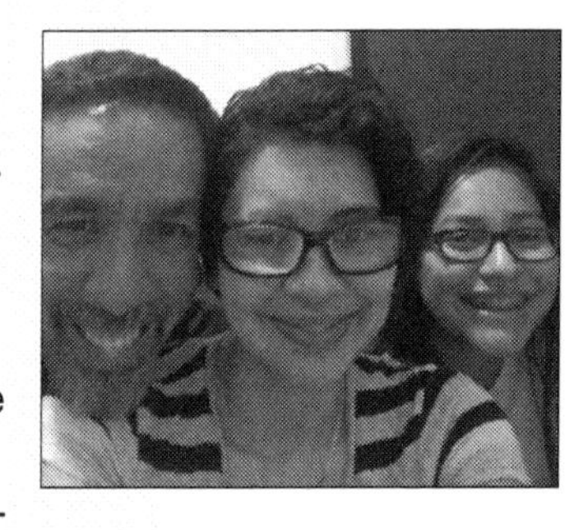

Editor's Note:
Ivy was told she was going to die because her cancer was so aggressive and conventional therapies offered very little confidence. She never lost faith or gave up hope, putting the power of prayer and her love of medicine (she holds numerous degrees, including a Doctor of Medicine, a PhD in biomedical and veterinary sciences, an MPH in health education and BSN in nursing) to work – discovering alternative and holistic strategies. Today, she remains cancer-free and is on mission to help others, even leading the very first Spanish speaking HealingStrong™ community group. You can locate her in Falls Church, VA through the HealingStrong™ group maps page: **www.healingstrong.org/groups**

I have a very broad medical and public health background and have worked on chronic disease prevention and control for the past 14 years. While I almost exclusively believed in traditional western medicine, I had some awareness that the environment and stress can influence our health. My ignorance made me think that I was well prepared to deal with any medical circumstance. However, I did not realize or appreciate how alternative medicine, lifestyle, and spiritual/emotional health can help one to reverse cancer.

My beliefs were shaken a year ago when I was told that I had Adenoid Cystic Carcinoma of the Lacrimal gland. Faced with the realization that chemotherapy and traditional radiation provide little hope against this type of cancer (and most any type of cancer), I suddenly felt helpless and vulnerable. And it wasn't until I finally got on my knees and prayed to God for mercy, that a human angel reached out to me. Seeing a Facebook post by "coincidence", my angel (who was also diagnosed about 6 years ago with the same kind of cancer) reached out and told me about Proton Radiation. Thanks to this information, I discovered the control of disease (prevention of recurrence) increased with this treatment.

Still, this was not enough. I needed to prevent metastasis. Through my conversations with "my angel" and my own research, I began to discover the dramatic benefits of holistic treatment. Through my prayer group, The Truth About Cancer website, Chris Wark, Kris Carr, Anita Moorjanil, and many friends, I learned that cancer is a complex disease that needs a complex approach. I came to understand how God's healing resources can be tapped into and used to recover. By engaging in a life transforming approach to diet, meditation, exercise, prayer, and forgiveness, my body and spirit began to detoxify itself from the physical and psycho-spiritual toxins that I didn't know I carried.

One year later, and my MRIs have remained completely clean. There have been no signs of any recurrence; I have faith that God will help me to stay cancer free. My life wasn't just saved by God; I was renewed and given a new life. I now want to share my experiences with those who are on the same path. HealingStrong offers a God's centered holistic approach and provides people like myself the opportunity to share our experiences and knowledge with those who are on the same path.

"Give your hand to serve, and your heart to love."

– Mother Teresa

TESTIMONIAL

JARED BUCEY

Hodgkin's Lymphoma Stage 4 (diagnosed at 16 years old)

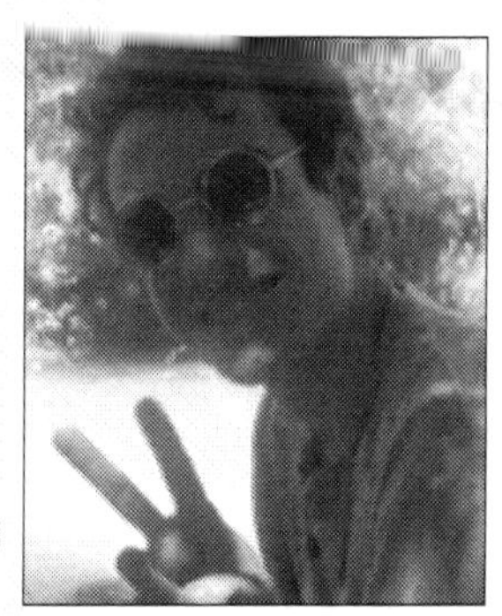

I was born with a rare heart defect called Hypoplastic Left Heart Syndrome and had a heart transplant when I was only four months old. In the summer of 2014, at the age of 16, I was diagnosed with stage four Hodgkin's lymphoma and given very little hope.

At that time, I knew what natural holistic treatment was at the time because my mom had been treating some very bad rashes using those techniques. Going through the diagnosis, I observed the other children who also had cancer and enduring a great deal of pain and suffering through the treatments. It was like a brotherhood and I felt their pain. The conventional chemotherapy seemed like the only option at the time. My feelings and gut intuition were telling me to do natural treatment while I was taking the chemo – but sadly, I had gotten so weak and sick from the chemo that I wasn't really able to do natural treatment alongside it, I just wasn't strong enough. Truth be told, I was barely alive after the first and only treatment. Within days of taking the chemo, I had sores all throughout my mouth and down my throat. I couldn't even eat from the pain it caused and my gums ended up swelling over my teeth! I also became very nauseous, my vision got very blurry and I wondered if I was going blind. I had extreme headaches and constant bone and muscle pain; I was practically paralyzed by the pain. I couldn't move without feeling sharp pain everywhere below my neck. When they gave me that dose of chemo, the person giving it to me was practically wearing a hazmat suit and had on a helmet that resembled a gas mask. When I asked why she was wearing all that she said she had to protect herself from the chemo and that she couldn't breathe it in or get it on her.

That's when it all came together for me and I began to question things... I still went through with it – for the other children who were being treated with chemo. After the extreme physical reaction that my body experienced, I was looking for a different way. I was inspired by Chris Wark of Chrisbeatcancer.com who encouraged me to change my internal terrain. I took countless supplements and vitamins, sat in an infrared sauna for a half hour to detox, jumped on a rebounder, went on nature walks, juiced raw organic vegetables, meditated every day and of course switched to eating all organic. As a direct result from this change, I've been cancer free for almost three years and continue to thrive with a natural holistic lifestyle. I started a popular Facebook page: Kid Against Chemo, and I just finished my autobiography a couple months ago and am about to move out on my own with dear friends. If there is anything I could say to help others it would be this, based on my own experience: I'd recommend eating all organic, eating very little meat if any, and I personally feel every illness stems from an emotional and/or spiritual illness. If you're sick in any way whatsoever, check your emotional and spiritual health as well as addressing the physical needs.

Editor's Notes:
For more of Jared's story, read a great interview here: **https://greenlivingaz.com/kid-against-chemo-update**.
Jared's Mom Lisa runs a HealingStrong™ Group in Cornville, AZ. For more information about this group or others, go to the map here and find the group: **www.healingstrong.org/groups**

A peaceful heart leads to a healthy body;
jealousy is like cancer in the bones.
– **Proverbs 14:30** *(NLT)*

For as he thinks in his heart, so is he.
– **Proverbs 23:7** *(NKJV)*

Aha! Moment #4
Sugar Feeds Cancer

> "Cancer cells have been long known to have a "sweet tooth," using vast amounts of glucose for energy and for building blocks for cell replication,"
>
> – **Johns Hopkins Medical Center**

One of the first things I was told I needed to do when I was diagnosed with cancer was to give up the sugar. For me, this was not an easy notion to accept. I needed to understand the science behind it before giving up my coveted Cokes, cookies and chocolate pie.

According to an article in Science Daily (August 18, 2009), researchers at Huntsman Cancer Institute at the University of Utah have uncovered new information on the notion that sugar "feeds" tumors. (For the full article go to: http://www.sciencedaily.com/releases/2009/08/090817184539.htm)

Cancer metabolizes through a process of fermentation. If you've ever made wine, you'll know that fermentation requires sugar. Sugars are the most common biochemistry of fermentation.

The metabolism of cancer is approximately eight times greater than the metabolism of normal cells.

Knowing the above, the body is constantly overworked trying to feed this cancer. The cancer is constantly on the verge of starvation and thus it is constantly asking the body to feed it. When the food supply is cut off, the cancer begins to starve unless it can make the body produce sugar to feed itself.

The wasting syndrome, cachexia, is the body producing sugar from proteins (you heard it right, not from carbohydrates or fats, but from proteins) in a process called glycogenesis. This sugar feeds the cancer. The body finally dies of starvation, trying to feed the cancer.

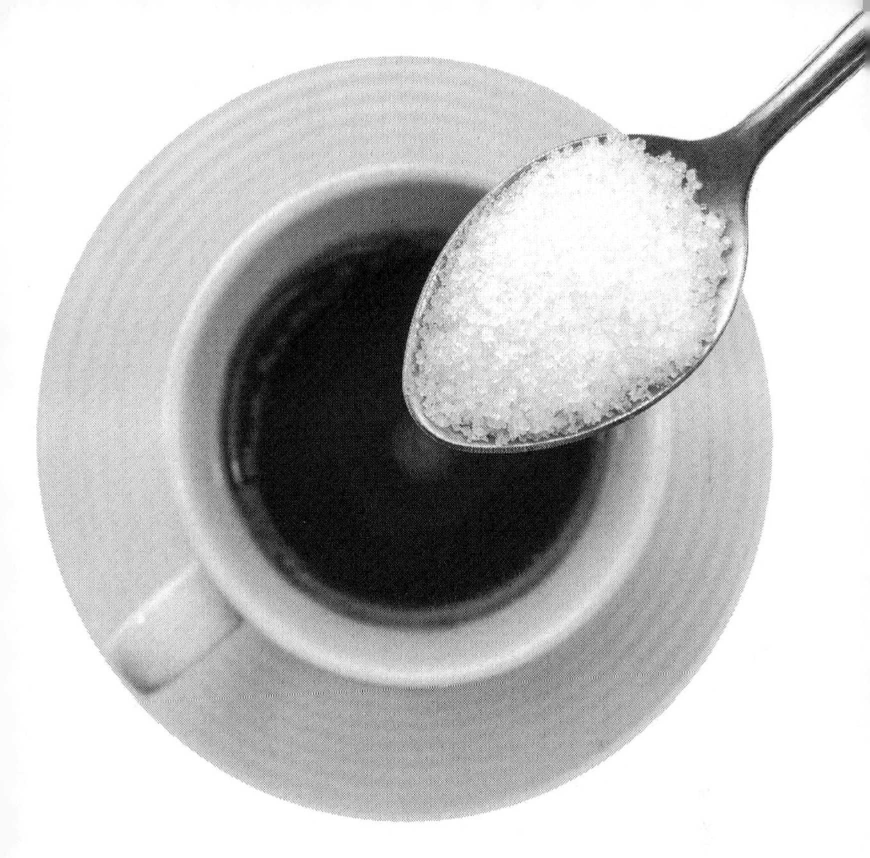

Now, knowing that one's cancer needs sugar, does it make sense to feed it sugar? Does it make sense to have a high carbohydrate diet? NO

The reason food therapies for cancer even exist today (beyond the fact that they work) is because someone once saw the connection between sugar and cancer. The therapeutic strategy of modifying the diet and eliminating sugar was definitely a principle form of therapy to healing strong.

There are many food therapies, but not a single one allows many foods high in carbohydrates and not a single one allows sugars, because sugar feeds cancer. Easy change…remove the fuel for the cancer cell, and increase my chances for beating cancer.

It was yet another Aha! Moment, resulting in a change that I implemented right away.

TESTIMONIAL

CORTNEY CAMPBELL

Nodular Lymphocyte Predominant Hodgkin's Lymphoma Stage 2

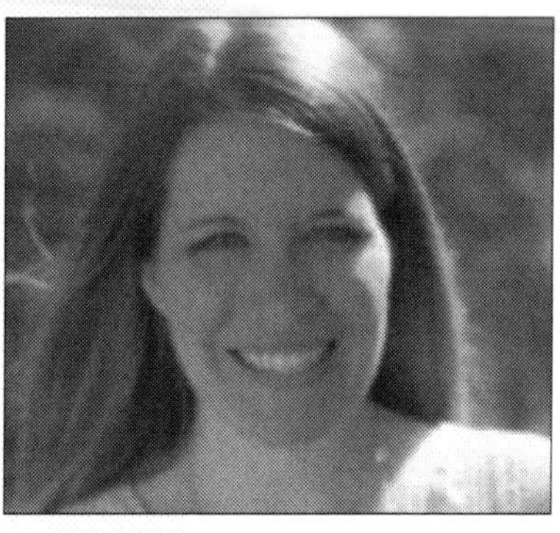

In the Fall of 2004 I found a lump in my neck. Knowing that my mom's twin sister had Hodgkin's Lymphoma as a teen, I was left very concerned. It was examined, an MRI was done, and I was given the option for a biopsy. I opted to withhold doing that for financial reasons – being a new college graduate with limited funds, instead I was given antibiotics and the lump shrunk temporarily.

In September of 2008, almost 4 years after my initial discovery of my neck's enlarged "cervical" lymph node, I found a new lump - this time in my right armpit. About a week later, I was in the general practitioner's office and within an hour I was getting lab work, then immediately sent to Piedmont Hospital in Atlanta for a consultation with a surgeon. He scheduled me for a full lumpectomy/ biopsy the very next day.

The results showed that it was a slow moving Hodgkin's Lymphoma with an excellent prognosis. The recommended treatment was three months (four cycles) of R-CHOP chemotherapy and radiation. They explained to me the side effects of this conventional therapy including: hair loss, nausea, mouth sores, and INFERTILITY. My first oncologist scheduled me for a CT/PET scan to confirm the suspected Stage II diagnosis, along with a bone marrow biopsy.

Over the next few weeks I did both, and both came back confirming my diagnosis of Stage II Nodular Lymphocyte Predominant Hodgkin's Lymphoma.

While I was awaiting my impending doom of chemotherapy and mourning the loss of my future children, my husband (of just 3 months), Kevin, began researching alternative cancer treatments. Kevin came in contact with was a man named Jerry Brunetti. Jerry healed his Stage 3 Non-Hodgkin Lymphoma with nutritional therapies and in an online presentation, he presented the individual healing powers of the food he consumed while healing. It made so much sense to us. Kevin also began ordering different books on alternative cancer protocols. One of these was Bill Henderson's Cancer-Free: Your Guide to Non-Toxic Healing. He shared stories of people who cured their cancer naturally. I really struggled with the idea of this because how could this "natural" treatment be so effective, yet doctors continue to treat almost exclusively with chemotherapy, radiation, and surgery? On November 4th I began a strict regimen of 2/3 cup organic cottage cheese and 6 tablespoons of flaxseed oil for breakfast every morning, a series of vitamins and supplements, and an immune booster made mainly from baker's yeast called Beta Glucan. My diet was strictly raw vegetables and juices. I even limited fruit to 2 servings per day. No sugar, meat, caffeine, processed foods, or cooked food.

December brought a new discovery – the Living Foods Institute in Atlanta. I was introduced to new ways to enjoy raw foods which help me cope with the depression that comes with such a drastic diet change. At the Living Foods Institute I received seven colonics to detox my colon. I say I was in "perfect health" before my diagnosis, but the truth is I had a SAD diet (Standard American Diet) of eating habits. My body was starving for nutrients. This is what I believe to be the main cause of my cancer. During this time we found out about Ty Bollinger's book: "Cancer: Step Outside the Box". In it we found reassurance that what we were doing was

God's plan for my healing. I began drinking Essiac tea as another weapon against the lymphoma, it was this that really detoxified my lymph system. We also bought an Alkaline Water Ionizer and all of the kitchen supplies we needed to prepare "Living" Foods. I had never sprouted a thing in my life and now I was sprouting wheatgrass, lentils, and mung beans and juicing wheatgrass every morning! I also began HcG Testing, a much cheaper and easy way to monitor the cancer. I began this in November and took a follow up in January right before the Living Foods Institute. I dropped almost an entire point in my score which was excellent progress.

Also, exercise and detoxification was important so we bought a Cellerciser rebounder. During this process my husband, myself, and my doctors kept physical track of the cancerous lymph node in my neck. At the next oncologist's visit my doctor couldn't even find the lump. I was scheduled to take my next HcG test in March. But instead I found out I was pregnant, we knew there was a chance of this since I had gone off all prescription medication, including birth control. I even had an OBGYN who refused to take me as a patient because "I refused to treat my cancer." I was treating my cancer, and it was working. The pregnancy made a situation that was difficult to begin with even harder. The importance of positive and prayerful thinking became even more relevant.

Through March and April we waited. I also could no longer monitor the cancer through HcG testing since human fetuses have high levels of HcG. It was an extremely tense time for our family. Shortly after, my oncologist gave us the incredible news that I was in remission. May 4th, 2009 I was declared in "clinical" remission. I have had a clean bill of health since then. I continue to be monitored via bloodwork and physical examinations. I went on to have an unmedicated and natural birth to Ruby-Claire Campbell on November 19th 2009. She is truly a miracle! As of this writing I am still in clinical remission and now we have two additional children to our family. I limit sugar and processed foods, and still rarely eat meat. When I do, it is grass fed, free-range meat or wild-caught fish. I eat a ton of nutrient-dense, organic vegetables every day and I still drink green tea and take 26 purposeful vitamin supplements a day.

For my husband and I, it was a prayerful decision to approach the cancer the way we did. We believe that God gave us a fully functioning, self-healing body that when brought back to its original state can fight off malfunctioning cell growth like cancer. It will be a journey to keep the cancer away, not a destination and I hope I can be an inspiration to encourage this belief.

My recommended resources include:

Cancer: Think Outside the Box by Ty Bollinger

Cancer-Free: Your Guide to Non-Toxic Healing by Bill Henderson

"Therefore once more I will astound these people with wonder upon wonder; the wisdom of the wise will perish, the intelligence of the intelligent will vanish."

Editor's Note:

Cortney shares her journey and wisdom in a popular blog that reaches thousands of people each month: **www.anticancermom.com**

She and her husband, Kevin, are also founding team members for HealingStrong™ and serve on the Board of Directors. A video of Cortney and Kevin can be seen here on the Truth About Cancer: Quest for the Cure: **https://thetruthaboutcancer.com/survivor-story-cortney-campbell**.

Another great video: **https://www.youtube.com/watch?v=cb3wA1vQnXs**

TESTIMONIAL

DANNY HARTHAN

Colon Cancer Stage 3
HealingStrong™ Group Leader
Charlotte, NC

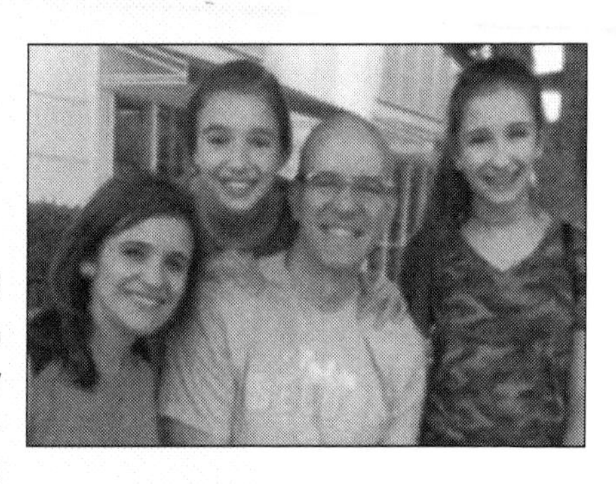

In December of 2012 I was diagnosed with colon cancer and was quickly scheduled for a colon resection in January of 2013 due to blockage created by the tumor. All of the scans prior to the surgery indicated that the cancer was contained to the colon. However, the pathology following the surgery revealed that it was Stage 3, metastasis in 10 of the 23 lymph nodes. The next week, my wife and I went to the oncologist's office for orientation. I signed all the forms stating that I understood the severe side effects from the chemotherapy. A couple of weeks later, when we went back again, I had two-pages of questions. The oncologist was very gracious and answered all of them. I was about to leave the office when one more question popped into my head. I asked: Does it matter what I eat? Should I be trying to eat really healthy… like lots of blueberries? At the time, blueberries were the healthiest thing that I was aware of so I asked if eating them in excess would help. He told me that I was allowed to eat whatever I wanted but maybe shouldn't eat an excessive amount of blueberries because they were antioxidants. He said they trying to kill cells and things like that will essentially neutralize some of the medicine. OK, thank you, I said – and that was that.

For me, it was a combination of several events that tipped the balance to create my own Aha moment. The first event happened shortly after I got home. I was unsettled and started thinking more about his answer to that last question. Surely he had misspoken – he must have meant to specify that we are trying to kill cancer cells... not just cells. Google can clear this up, I thought... "what does chemotherapy kill?" What???? Unfortunately, chemotherapy does not know the difference between cancer cells and the normal cells. This was alarming to me and I really didn't know what to do with this information.

I wasn't aware of anything, and no one in my circle of friends ever mentioned anything to me other than chemotherapy. The more I read about chemotherapy, the more I realized that the potential side effects I had signed off on weren't to be taken lightly... like the way I ignore the voice overs on the TV commercials about side effects of different prescription medications. One of them that I had signed off on could cause leukemia down the road. I clearly remember thinking "There has to be something better than this. This is worse than Russian roulette – there is a bullet in every chamber. I'll be poisoning myself with every round." Back to Google. What I would term my second event was actually a series of discoveries over the course of the next several days: 1) Dr. Otto Warburg's discovery that sugar is the fuel of cancer cells, 2) everyone has cancer cells in their body, and 3) your immune system is responsible for killing cancer cells. All of the research around these facts were eye opening and added to my arsenal of information and tools I needed to make an informed decision. I started looking into 1) diets low in sugar, 2) ways to build a super immune system, and 3) natural treatments for cancer.

I also went looking for advice from people I trust who were mindful of health and wellness. I called a friend of mine who I knew had recently made a big shift towards a healthy lifestyle and asked him for advice. He invited me to a seminar that his chiropractor was having in a few days about health and this same sort of healthy lifestyle that I was asking about. Figuring I didn't have anything to lose, my wife and I went and listened and the picture was starting to come into focus and the balance continued to move towards non-toxic treatments. Ironically, shortly after my surgery, a family friend (the wife of a conventional doctor) came over to visit. She said something to the effect of, "Make sure you finish all the rounds of chemo. And don't let any chiropractor talk you out of it." At the time, that seemed like a silly thing to say. Noone was going to talk me out of chemo. I was seeking wisdom and looking for understanding.

The next domino to fall was the book The Cancer Killers. It is the story of Dr. Charles Majors who, after being diagnosed with multiple myeloma, was given weeks to live. He embarked on a healing journey using all holistic, non-medical interventions. He was proclaimed to be cancer-free at the five-year anniversary of his diagnosis after an MRI revealed no tumors in Dr. Charles' brain. Despite these events continuing to tip the balance towards non-toxic therapies, I was still not totally convinced to forego chemo. It was a difficult choice, when I told people that I was considering alternative medicine, they either told me they didn't agree with it or you could see the disapproval on their face. I postponed my chemo treatment for three weeks in a row – each time with a little more pushback from the oncologist's office. They kept telling me it was essential to get started because it was a fast moving cancer and spreading more each day. I still had no peace and kept researching.

One day, Chris Wark's website (chrisbeatcancer.com) showed up in one of my Google searches. Finally, I found a connection with someone current that had lived this cancer, and had been successful. At that time, it was before Chris' online Square One program was available; he would offer personal consultations with people. I actually spoke with him and gained a tremendous amount of insight and peace of mind. That was the last piece of my puzzle. The conversation with Chris, along with all the other events made my decision crystal clear. I called up the office and told them that I was actually not going do the chemo. Within five minutes, the oncologist called me back on my cell phone exhorting me to think about my kids and wife. He told me that I was essentially signing my death warrant and that there was no way that the surgery had gotten all of the cancer – not with metastasis in 10 of the 23 lymph nodes. He told me that my chances of survival without chemo were only 40%. Yet, I felt confident that I was on the right path.

Isaiah 40:31 (NIV)

But those who hope in the LORD will renew their strength. They will soar on wings like eagles; they will run and not grow weary, they will walk and not be faint.

In Apr. 2013, I started under the care of a naturopath in Memphis, TN. In order to combat my cancer, I did everything I could. This included: far infrared sauna, vitamin-C IV, hydrocolonics, apricot kernels, a LOT of supplements, removed all the amalgam fillings with a holistic dentist, herbal tinctures, chiropractic care, coffee enemas, colon cleanses, liver cleanses, Big Berkey water filter, shower filters, hyperbaric oxygen chamber, rebounding, exercise, got rid of all the lawn chemicals, stopped using a lawn service to spray for weeds, stopped using the pest company to spray in and around the house, eliminated all processed sugar, gluten, dairy, and meat from my diet and switched to an organic, plant based diet, got rid of our microwave, switched to non-toxic, non-chemical cleaning products, a LOT of juicing, and essential oils. Slowly the markers began improving. I had a PET scan in Oct. 2013 and it came back completely cancer-free. I became aware of HealingStrong™ after watching Chris Wark's Square One modules. HealingStrong™ seemed like a perfect fit for me to be able to connect with others and try to help encourage those trying to navigate a similar path to mine. I want to be able to connect and help others , as a fellow survivor, like Chris did for me.

My favorite resources to recommend are:

- cancertutor.com
- naturalnews.com
- thetruthaboutcancer.com
- chrisbeatcancer.com
- anticancermom.com
- breastcancerconqueror.com
- greenmedinfo.com
- Chris Wark's Square One Program: sn188.infusionsoft.com/go/go/HealingStrong

To locate Danny's HealingStrong™ group in Charlotte, NC, or others like it: **www.healingstrong.org/groups**

TESTIMONIAL

DAVID LINGLE

Chronic
Lymphocytic Leukemia
HealingStrong™
Group Leader
Salisbury, NC

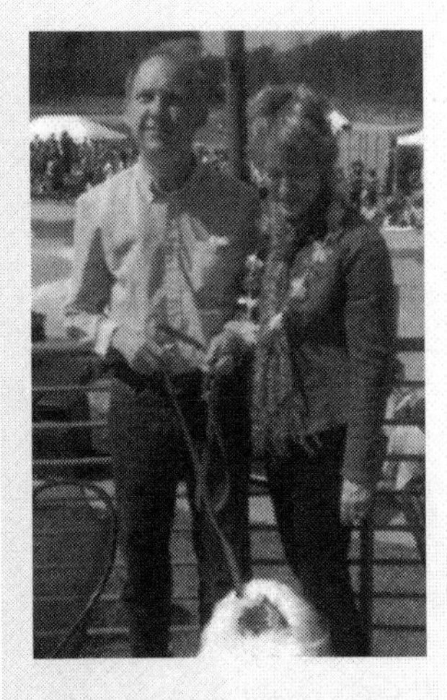

In October 2011, I was diagnosed with CLL (chronic lymphocytic leukemia) after a routine blood work came back and my white blood cell count was 52,000. A bone marrow biopsy confirmed it. I came home that same day, cleaned the kitchen out of ALL processed foods and told Brenda, my wife, that I was going raw vegan.

Brenda had been researching natural healing for the body for a number of years and being a Type 1 diabetic for 40 years, we knew that steroids, chemo and radiation were not good options. My personal journey to healing began and I never doubted that I was going to beat CLL naturally – and I never looked back.

During my healing journey, I started by doing a colon, liver and kidney cleanse because if your colon isn't clean, your body cannot absorb the nutrients needed to heal. I would start my day each day and thanking God for another day and His healing. I checked my pH daily and keep it between 7 and 7.4 using Biotech TriSalts, baking soda or Organic Braggs Apple Cider Vinegar. Cancer has a hard time surviving in an alkaline body. I also took 4 Maitake D Fraction Mushroom capsules to build up my immune system, along with a number of other supplements. My breakfast consisted of a Budwig protocol serving of Budwig's flax oil and cottage cheese with blueberries and ground flax seeds. I also consumed green drinks including: Dr. Schulze's Superfood Plus, barley grass powder, chlorella powder, astragalus and dandelion root powder, and One World Whey Powder. The astragalus root powder, an adaptogen, helped me to build my immune system while the dandelion is specific to my blood related cancer. I also drink 3 ounces of Essaic Tea and Dr. Mercola's recipe for turmeric powder with a teaspoon of organic coconut oil. I also made sure to take probiotics daily. As for other meals, lunch consisted of a green smoothie and supper, a large salad and maybe some cooked veggies with organic pasta, brown rice or quinoa.

In addition to all of this, I focused on drinking veggie juices each day, along with four barley grass drinks in between. Keeping my body hydrated is key, and these super green drinks increase oxygen to the body. I was sure to drink half my bodyweight in ounces of clean filtered water a day. I have learned along the way that exercise is another very important element to help build the immune system and my use of a FIR (far infrared) sauna two to three times weekly can help remove toxins that build up. I also have had ALL mercury removed and three of five root canal teeth removed because of the harmful effects mercury has on the human body.

In August 2013 I was informed the CLL was gone per an ONCO-blot test done by my integrative MD. After two years of a holistic healing approach I was able to recapture my life again, stronger than ever before.

Today to maintain my health, I continue to eat organic raw foods and drink a 32 ounce green smoothie. I juice on occasions but not daily and also occasionally will eat small amounts of organic grass fed bison, chicken, and wild caught salmon. Most of the rest of my diet changes have remained intact. I've learned that besides eating healthy and juicing, it is very important to believe in yourself and know that you can heal. I also have found a key element to healing is to get rid of the internal baggage that has setup shop. We all carry something that we have held onto from past experiences, and this can hinder one's ability to heal. Get rid of it.

I highly recommend these books to people who are interested in learning more about a holistic approach:
Cancer: Think Outside the Box by Ty Bollinger
Killing Cancer - Not People by Robert Wright

Editor's Note:
For more information about David's healing journey, here is a great video testimonial and write up: **www.chrisbeatcancer.com/david-refused-chemo-and-healed-leukemia-naturally**

To locate David's HealingStrong™ group in Salisbury, NC, or others like his – go to the map and find the location you are interested at: **www.healingstrong.org/groups**

Verses of encouragement:

"Come to Me, all you who labor and are heavy laden, and I will give you rest. Take My yoke upon you and learn from Me, for I am gentle and lowly in heart, and you will find rest for your souls. For My yoke is easy and My burden is light."
– Matthew 11:28:30

Aha! Moment #5
Oxygen Fights Cancer

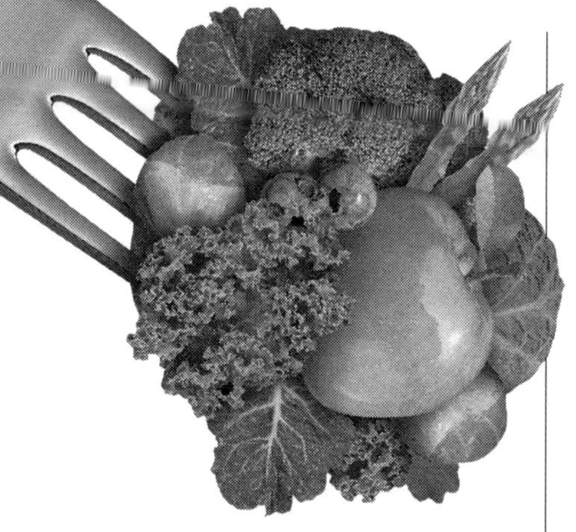

TYPES OF OXYGEN THERAPY

There are two types of oxygen therapies readily available in many holistic clinics:

- Ozone or O3 (3 oxygen atoms) and forms an energetic molecule that donates it's third oxygen atom to free radicals which cause damage to our bodies through oxidation.
- Hyperbaric chambers flood tissue and vital organs with oxygen at the cellular level by incorporating pressurized ambient air to dissolve oxygen directly into the plasma, cerebral and spinal fluids, flooding tissues and vital organs with oxygen

After starting with the removal of sugar from my diet, I kept coming across information about the importance of keeping my body's biochemistry at an alkaline state. An important Aha! Moment came when I understood the basic biochemistry and how changes affect my overall health.

The International Wellness Directory explains that Otto Warburg discovered in the 1930's the main biochemical cause of cancer, or what differentiates a cancer cell from a normal, healthy cell. This discovery was so significant that Otto Warburg was awarded the Nobel Prize.

His discovery tells us that cancer metabolizes much differently than normal cells. Normal cells need oxygen. Cancer cells despise oxygen. In fact, oxygen therapy is a favorite among many of the alternative clinics I've researched.

The foods I would eat actually caused a chain reaction. Acid-forming foods, carbohydrates such as donuts, candy, milk shakes, ice cream, soda, bread, pastries, etc., make the blood more acidic. The more acidic the blood is, the less oxygen it contains. Thus, the importance of lowering carbohydrate intake and keeping the body at an alkaline state. Placing foods into an acid vs. alkaline chart made sense to me.

Understanding the pH of our bodies in relation to health is important to understanding the totality of disease and reversing its effects.

Our arterial or urine pH is an indicator of health and wellness. PH or potential of hydrogen, is a measurement used to determine the acidity or alkalinity of a liquid. pH is important to our health since our bodies are mostly made up of liquids.

The pH scale goes from 0 to 14, while 7 is neutral. Below 7 is acidic, and above 7 is alkaline. The body's design is to be around 7.4. When it falls below this, the body becomes acidic and health problems can occur. The lower the number the more acidic. Cancerous tissues are acidic, whereas healthy tissues are alkaline. At a pH slightly above 7.4 cancer cells become dormant and at pH 8.5 cancer cells will die while healthy cells will live (Robert R. Barefoot & Carol J. Reich, M.D., The Scientific Secret of Health and Youth, 2002)

Interestingly, there's a major difference in oxygen even within the narrow range of "normal" blood pH: Blood that is pH 7.3 actually has 69.4% less oxygen than 7.45 blood, according to scientist Sang Whang's book, *Reverse Aging.*

So this means we should do everything to keep the pH on the high side of the range, as close as possible to 7.45, by eating as many alkaline foods as possible. (Dr Tim O'Shea in TO THE CANCER PATIENT
www.thedoctorwithin.com)

"Eating alkaline foods balances the pH of the blood, which, in turn, inhibits the proliferation of cancer cells. Alkaline foods keep the blood pH in its ideal range of between 7.2 and 7.4, which is important for the prevention and treatment of cancer. Ideally, the diet should consist of 80 percent alkalineforming foods, such as those available from many raw fruits and vegetables, as well as nuts, seeds, grains, and legumes."

– **Gary Null, PhD**
In *The Complete Encyclopedia of Natural Healing,* 2005

"It is necessary to remove excess acidity and toxic chemicals from the body before health can be restored. To remove excess acidity from the tissues it is necessary to build up a reserve of alkalinity through an alkaline (vegan/mostly raw foods) diet, supplemented with fresh fruit and vegetable juices and alkaline minerals. Then this alkalinity must be moved around the body by any technique that works," Null says.

In addition to taking in a more alkaline diet, detoxification methods may be used for moving acidic or toxic materials out of the body in order to regenerate health. The Gerson diet uses a method of detoxing the body that is proven to be very effective (www.gerson.org). According to Alkalize for Health, vigorous exercise such as on the rebound mini-trampoline is reported to increase lymph flow by

15 to 30 times, which detoxifies and adds cancer-fighting oxygen to the body.

Learning the role that oxygen and pH levels play in fighting cancer was a big Aha! Moment for me, especially when I realized that there were ways I could actually change my body's biochemistry to fight the cancer process!

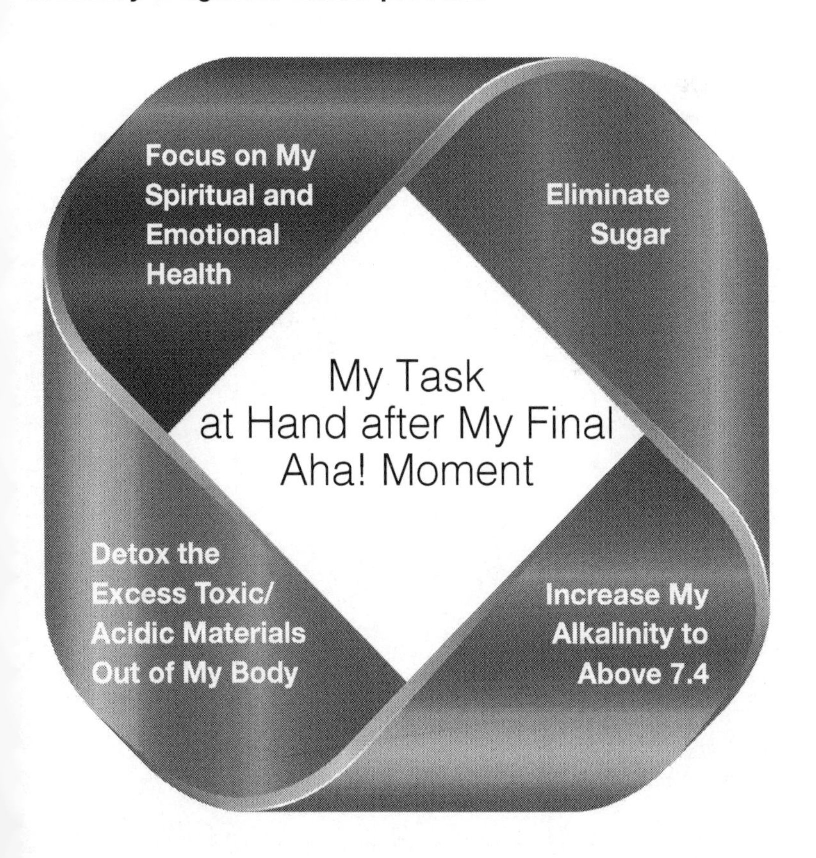

TESTIMONIAL

A Special Group of Breast Cancer Thrivers

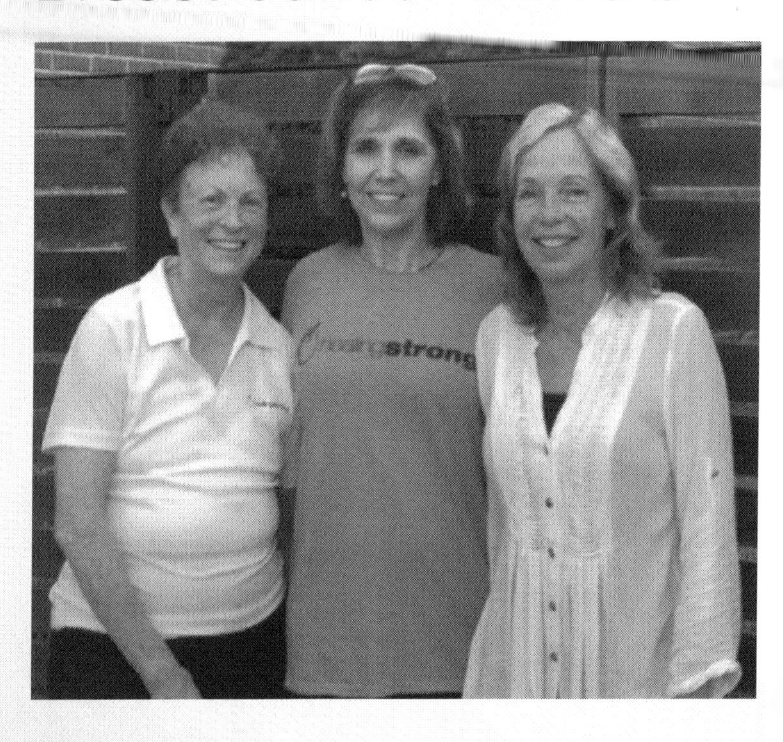

"My children, our love should not be just words and talk; it must be true love, which shows itself in action."

– 1 John 3:18 (GNT)

In September 2013, we wrapped up our first HealingStrong™ Conference. It was evident to the team that bringing people together, encouraging, praying for and with them, and sharing hope was mission critical. People need to be seen, heard and encouraged in person. After the conference, calls and emails poured in from people who wanted to continue to meet together. One of those people was Christine Holcomb, a conference attendee and breast cancer thriver. She expressed the desire to carry on what was started at the conference.

The HealingStrong™ atmosphere was different than any other traditional cancer conferences or groups she had attended. Her sentiments were shared by many. It didn't matter what people were facing, participants, spoke of the love they experienced, and walked away empowered with hope. They desired meaningful connections with those using holistic strategies to heal strong, with God at the center. They wanted to continue to learn through their journey, connecting and sharing hope with others. Christine and two of her friends, Marsha and Lynn, who also attended the conference, started their own HealingStrong™ group – meeting every month in their hometown. Their group has grown in the last 4 years, hosting world renowned authors and speakers at their monthly event, such as Dr. Veronique Desaulniers, Brenda Stockdale, and Dr. Eric Zielinski. They have helped organize local holistic conferences and events that have helped to educate and encourage thousands. Their effort and commitment to grow community centered on true health of mind, body and soul set the model for other HealingStrong™ Groups around the world today. Their personal dedication to help others and their stories of healing are an inspiration to me. I wanted to introduce you to these three amazing ladies.

TESTIMONIAL

CHRISTINE HOLCOMB

Breast Cancer
Stage 2
HealingStrong™
Group Leader
Gainesville, GA

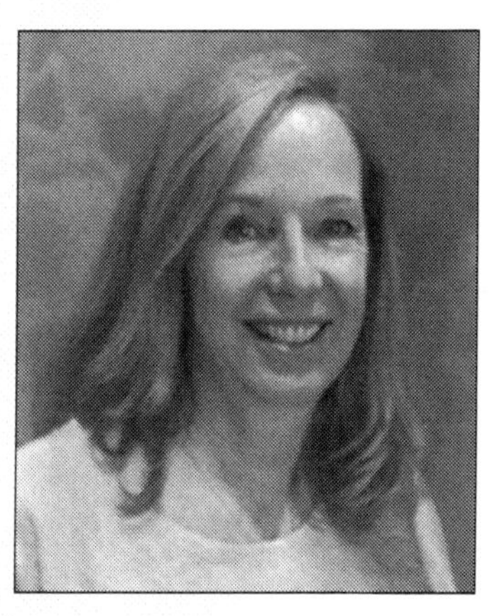

"Healing is a return to Love"
– Marianne Williamson

I had felt the lump for two years. The mammograms were clear and even my OB thought the lump was nothing. We finally saw it with the ultrasound, finding out the results of my biopsy hit me with titanic force. And so began my journey. My whole family was shaken by the news. I thought I was the healthy one and the questions "how?" and "why?" were repeating on an endless cycle in my head.

I was diagnosed with stage 2-ER+, PR+, and HER-, Ductal and Lobular carcinoma. Breast cancer. For years, I was the one that had walked in all the cancer walks, raised funds, organized teams for everyone else, now it was my turn to help myself.

After getting over the shock, I immediately had two surgeries in the following six months, which included a mastectomy.

The oncologist and my surgeon wanted me on Aromatase inhibitors… but I started reading at that point and decided I could get rid of the bad estrogens and balance my hormones. I began researching what makes our cells healthy and what makes things go wrong. I did try the chemicals for a few months because my surgeon begged me and he was chief of surgery at Emory. It was hard to go against him, but after studying the web, books, articles, talking to alternative doctors, and lots of prayer, I slowly began changing the way I ate.

After reading extensively, I realized that even though I had a fairly good diet, I was a sugar addict. I also took hormones for years, including birth control pills, used pesticides, used chemicals daily on my body, and ate processed and sprayed food. In addition to this I had lots of mercury in my teeth fillings and harbored resentments for long periods of time. It was time to change all of that.

Since my diagnosis, I now avoid genetically modified, chemically sprayed, and processed foods. I eat as fresh and clean as I can. I have gone from all raw while detoxing to eating some clean meat once in a while. I take some supplements, especially enzymes and probiotics. I juice regularly and make lots of green smoothies with sprouts. I believe that we can block or increase our own energy and healing by what we eat, think, or say. I have also taken up yoga. It helps me quiet myself, be still, and know HE is there! Recently I found that because of a mutation in my MTHFR gene I do not methylate well, so I'm supplementing to adjust. I am also volunteering with HealingStrong™, helping to lead the first "patient to patient" group in North metro Atlanta area to help others believe and understand about using natural methods to support healing.

While no one wants to hear they have cancer, I was nourished because of this diagnosis. I have watched so many family members change their life habits for the better and today, I feel better than I have in years. From a medical standpoint, everything you eat, drink, and breath affects our cells... either good, or bad.

This journey has also helped me learn more about how to live life to the fullest. I now know to forgive quickly as grudges never help a situation. I also have learned to slow down to stop and smell the roses of life while finding what is truly important and not letting the little stuff bother you. Most importantly – love everyone.

Recommended Resources that Most Inspired my HealingStrong Journey:

- *Crazy Sexy Diet*
  by Chris Karr
- *The Makers Diet*
  by Jordan Rubin
- *Empty Harvest*
  by Dr. Bernard Jenson
- *Healing the Gerson Way*
  by Charlotte Gerson
- *You can Beat the Odds*
  by Brenda Stockdale
- *The Iodine Crisis*
  by Lynne Farrow
- *Evaluating Alternative Cancer Therapies*
  by David Hess PHD
- *Cellular Awakening*
  by Barbara Wren
- *Heal Breast Cancer Naturally*
  by Dr. Veronique Desaulniers

TESTIMONIAL

LYNN KEARNS

Breast Cancer
HealingStrong™
Group Leader
Gainesville, GA

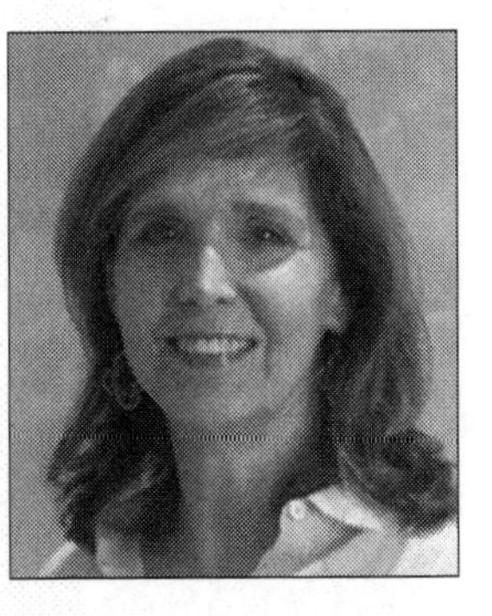

I was diagnosed with Invasive Ductal Carcinoma, stage one, in November of 2009. A month later I endured a lumpectomy and Sentinel node biopsy. I had found a very small, painful superficial lump that past spring and immediately went for a mammogram. Mammogram was negative and the doctor said just watch it. Six months later, my gynecologist, who had just returned from her own breast cancer treatment, encouraged me to have a biopsy. I underwent 22 days of Canadian Fractionation Radiation. It was recommended that I have chemotherapy, followed by aromatase inhibitors for five years.

As a registered nurse and health practitioner, with an advanced degree in cell biology, I researched conventional and holistic strategies. I looked for the stories of success. I read a book that helped me to realize that I was responsible for a healthy terrain, *Anti-Cancer: A New Way of Life* by David Servin-Schreiber. My remarkably made body had communicated to me through the cancer that I needed to make some changes. I incorporated a holistic approach to healing that included: Budwig diet, smoothies, juices, removing all sugar and processsed foods, acupuncture, and an Ayurvedic detox. I also attended the Living Food Institute which provided me with knowledge of a

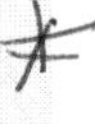

raw foods diet and detoxification strategies. Lastly, I used thermography instead of mammography to monitor my progress. I chose not to incorporate chemotherapy and radiation.

Finding real stories and real strategies gave me hope. I looked at the survivors that I knew who were thriving long-term, and none of them had taken chemotherapy. By taking this less known natural approach, I felt a bit like I was traveling alone through the wilderness, rejecting a great deal of conventional "wisdom".

The healing path is a very personal decision. If there is anything I would tell someone on a healing journey today, it's that you must trust your "gut" to make correct choices. Listen to that still small voice. Have faith. Don't let others push you off the path that you know deep in your soul is the correct one for you. Others may try to bully you, but stand up for your beliefs. I gained confidence as I studied the stories of success, and connected with others who were also on a similar path. Leading a local HealingStrong™ group provides me with confident assurance each month as I continue to connect and walk beside others on a healing journey.

TESTIMONIAL

MARSHA DICKEY

Throat and
Breast Cancer
HealingStrong™
Group Leader
Gainesville, GA

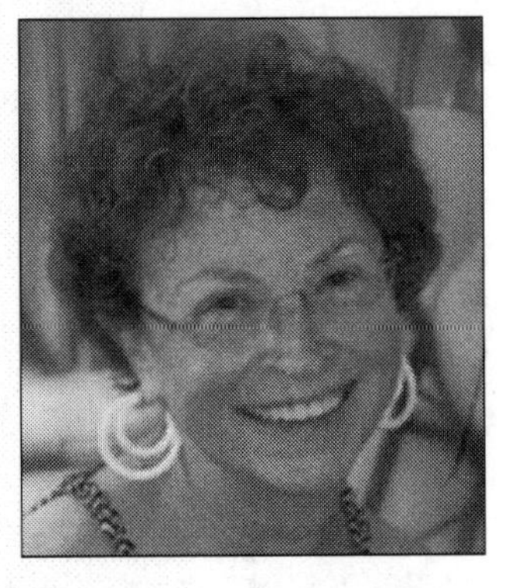

Since 2004, I have had two cancer diagnoses. What I have learned over these last many years has led me on a healing journey today that is very different then when I began. In September 2004, I was first diagnosed with throat cancer. I did what the doctors recommended and went through with the chemotherapy and radiation, which left me on a feeding tube. I began incorporating massive doses of Immune 26 in the feeding tube. After treatment, I had to learn how to swallow and eat, as my throat was so burned from the radiation. During that time, I asked the cancer nutritionist what to eat, and she told me to eat milkshakes and ice cream. This was off to me because I knew that sugar feeds cancer cells. In my mind, it was time to move on because clearly the nutritionist was lacking some very basic understanding of how cancer metabolizes.

After recovery, I went to Canyon Ranch for ten days and learned about clean eating and different alternative modalities.

In October 2008, I was diagnosed with cancer again, only this time it was breast cancer. I had a double mastectomy and afterwards I became a participant of a research project that used a product called Poly MVA along with several other natural substances. I then became a patient of Dr. Nicholas Gonzalez and Dr. Linda Issacs. I have been on this protocol for over four years. It encompasses diet, detoxification, and supplements designed specifically for me.

When I first was diagnosed with cancer, it was difficult to find any information about natural treatments but today there is an abundant amount of information on the internet and in books. HealingStrong™ offers a safe and supportive environment to learn about the options that support the body's ability to heal. HealingStrong™ is a community that lovingly shares information and supports your decision and gives you a hand to hold. It has become my own healing family.

Cancer is no longer a death sentence. For me, I stay positive and focus not only on the physical side of healing, but also on a spiritual place that supports my healing. Most of all – I am grateful for every day – even if it's "I brushed my teeth today." Research and talk to others who have experienced the cancer struggle. Begin with a HealingStrong™ group.

Helpful resources I have used include:

Ty Bollinger's Truth About Cancer series:
http://go.thetruthaboutcancer.rocks/?gl=582822956&a_aid=56034db58e51d&a_bid=e8f0d278

Knockout
by Suzanne Sommers

The Cancer Revolution
by Dr. Leigh Erin Connealy

Finding a HealingStrong™ connection at
www.healingstrong.org

Would you like to start a HealingStrong™ Group in your hometown? Please go to: www.healingstrong.org/groups and click: Start a Group.

You can also find information about existing groups on the map. All of our group leaders have knowledge of holistic strategies either as a patient, caregiver or practitioner.

For more information on their group, go to: **www.healingstrong.org/groups**

NEXT STEPS

After realizing my final Aha! Moment, my next task at hand was to:

- focus on my spiritual and emotional health;
- eliminate sugar;
- increase my alkalinity to above 7.4; and
- detox the excess toxic/acidic materials out of my body

My Aha! Moments helped to focus on what my plan needed to be and motivated me to approach my healing from a holistic perspective. I didn't "walk away" from treatment. My focus in healing strong was very intentional and determined, and included healing of the mind, body and spirit. It is a process and all three aspects of myself had to be addressed. While this book does not include the step-by-step process of everything I chose to do for 18 months to heal my cancer, I do include my dietary protocol in the pages to follow.

Recently, my friend, Chris Wark of Chris Beat Cancer released a coaching program (Square One) to help people through their journey to wellness using a non-toxic approach. Square One is one of the very best coaching programs I have seen. Chris's module on spiritual and emotional healing hits the nail on the head. I have seen so many people do all of the physical components to healing while ignoring the spiritual and emotional components. My experience, from my own life and observing others, tells me that in order to heal, one must address all three.

My prayer for you is that this little book will not be a stopping point, but rather a stepping stone to a pathway of healing strong and staying strong. Keep reading, searching, and most of all, ask God to show you His way, seeking His peace for the answer. If you don't have a peace about something, don't consent.

I hope that you will find the answers you are looking for and your journey to healing strong will be a life-giving experience. Connecting with others who are using natural therapies for healing would be a great starting point. You can find connections on our website at: www.healingstrong.org/groups.

About HealingStrong

HealingStrong™ creates community, encourages education and explores holistic methods for HealingStrong™ – mind, body, and soul. We engage healing of the mind through education to re-invigorate life and expectations. We engage healing of the body through emphasis on nutrition, detoxification, physical exercise, and holistic healing methods. We engage healing of the soul through encouraging emotional wholeness, and spiritual renewal with affirmations and promises from God's word.

HealingStrong™ Mission Statement
Our mission is to connect, support, and educate individuals facing cancer and other diseases with holistic, evidence-based non-toxic therapies. We believe that God created our bodies to be healthy, and that when His design of nutrition, exercise, emotional freedom, and spiritual peace is honored, then we can live in optimal health. We seek to walk in healing and to help others become HealingStrong™.

SUZY'S PERSONAL PERSPECTIVE

While all of my research showed that modern medicine wasn't adequately addressing the problem of cancer, and that a more natural approach including healthy dietary changes made more sense than adding poisonous chemicals to my body, I can't emphasize enough what an important role prayer and spirituality has played in my ability to heal strong.

Many scientific studies have shown the power of prayer in healing, and modern miracles take place every day. I am living proof of that. I believe in my heart that it was ultimately God who healed me, and my faith in His only son, the Lord Jesus Christ, sustained me through my healing journey.

At HealingStrong™, we recognize that it is easy to lose faith in the face of cancer. Nevertheless, we encourage you to believe that there is One who is more powerful than any cancer, and our stories give testimony to that. I pray that as you move through your own journey with cancer, you will find God's peace and experience His power to heal, as I have.

"For I am the Lord, who heals you."

Exodus 15:26

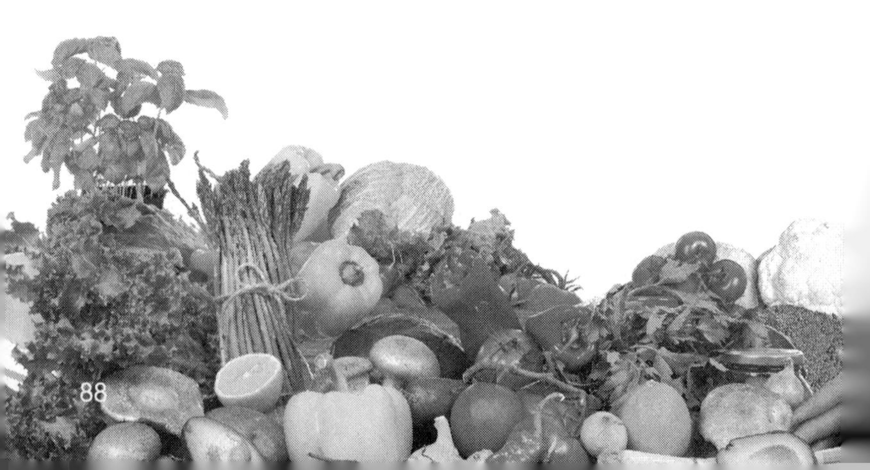

MY HEALING PROTOCOL

This is a general idea of a day in my healing journey. I was inspired by these books that really resonated with me and provided a "how to" game plan: *A Cancer Therapy: Results of Fifty Cases*, by Dr. Max Gerson, *Healing the Gerson Way* by Charlotte Gerson; and *My Cancer Battle Plan* by Anne Fraham. A resource for those interested in following a Gerson meal plan is the ***Gerson Therapy Handbook*** (found and printed here: http:// gerson.org/ pdfs/ GersonTherapyHandbook.pdf. Recipes start on page 102.) While I did modify some, the Gerson protocol has been well-documented and studied and should be closely followed. A sample of foods for the Gerson diet can be found here: https:// gerson.org/ pdfs/ Foods-For-The-Gerson-Diet.pdf.

My protocol followed a vegan diet with extensive juicing and detoxification, along with supplementation. I kept my meal plan simple and ate practically the same plant-based diet for breakfast and lunch, varying my dinners each night. My vegan diet was organic as much as possible with no sugar, no salt, no caffeine, no dairy, and no oils. I also drank between 8-10 fresh juices a day and did two to three detoxes each day.

IMPORTANT TO NOTE:
I followed my protocol for 18 months, and during that time, I would add various adjunct therapies, such as high doses of vitamin C powder, Essiac tea and apricot kernels. I wasn't consistent with the adjunct therapies, but adhered to the primary therapy shared below. (I do believe adjunct therapies can be beneficial to fighting cancer and other diseases.)

A DAY IN MY LIFE:

7:00 am FRESH JUICE:

6 ounce glass of fresh squeezed citrus juice (orange or grapefruit)

7:30/8:00 am BREAKFAST:

6-8 ounce glass of fresh carrot juice 3-4 carrots, 1 green apple) Large portion oatmeal (cut up green apple with cinna- mon); Bread (rye) toasted or plain

8:30 - 9:00 am LIVER DETOX:

Coffee Enema - See Lesson 4 for Resource Links. I used this "down time" to listen to scriptures either through YouVersion on my phone or a CD entitled *Heaven's Health Food* by Larry Hutton (healing scriptures set to music) https:// larryhutton.org/ product/heavens-health-food/.

9:30 am FRESH JUICE:

6-8 ounce glass of fresh green juice (handful of romaine lettuce, swiss chard, beet greens, green pepper (1/4 of small one) varying types of kale, 1/2 green apple

Supplementation:

Curcumin, cinnamon capsules, CoQ10, IP6 and Inositol, KyoGreen powder (I would often add this to my green drinks throughout the day), and Vitamin D3. I didn't take Iodine regularly during my healing journey (I didn't know about the importance of it until recently, but thanks to Lynne Farrow's book *The Iodine Crisis*, I do take it today) along with Beta-1, 3D Glucan. Most cancer patients are deficient and need adequate supplementation. The fresh fruits and vegetables on this protocol provided super nutrients, and the additional supplementation helped boost the fight for cancer and improve my immune function.

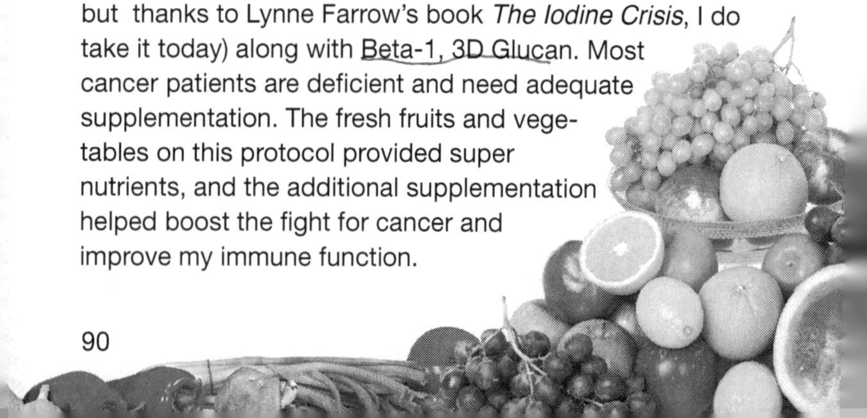

11:00 am **SNACK:**
Fruit with handful of raw almonds (not Gerson)
6-8 ounce glass of fresh carrot juice (recipe page 90)

12:00 pm **LIVER DETOX:**
Same as page 90.

12:30 pm **LUNCH:**
Baked potato seasoned with lemon juice and dried Italian organic seasonings. Large green salad with assortment of raw vegetables (broccoli, kale, spinach, green pepper, green lettuce, tomato, purple cabbage). Fresh juice - green and carrot juice (3 carrots, 1 green apple, 2 swiss chard leaves, 2 kale leaves, 1/2 lemon).

2:00 pm **FRESH JUICE:**
Fresh carrot juice (recipe page 90).

2:30 pm **NAP:**
I was blessed to have a job where I telecommuted and could schedule power naps in the day. I napped at least 30 minutes each day. Rest is an important part of healing strong.

3:30 pm **SNACK:**
Fresh raw vegetable or fruit (celery, cucumber, orange, 1/2 banana), or I would heat up a bowl of oatmeal with cut up apples and cinnamon.
Fresh Juice - green juice (recipe above).

6:00 pm DINNER:

Fresh Juice: 1/2 beet, 2 carrots, handful of spinach and kale, ½ lemon (not Gerson) Salad (all raw). Baked potato - seasoned with lemon juice and parsley, with stewed vegetables such as squash, zucchini, and onions (each day, my vegetables for supper varied, and I may have asparagus, cauliflower, broccoli or something else.)

Hippocrates Soup Recipe

For 1 person use a 4-quart pot with the following vegetables, then cover with filtered water (I have a Berkey Water Filter): 1 medium celery knob (substitute 3-4 stalks of celery), 1 medium parsley root, garlic as desired, 2 small leeks, 1-1/ 2 lbs. tomatoes or more, 2 medium onions, 1 lb. potatoes, a handful of parsley, and 2 cups of shredded cabbage. Do not peel any of these vegetables; just wash and scrub them well and cut them coarsely. Simmer them slowly for 2 hours, then put through food mill in small portions. Vary the amount of water used for cooking, according to taste and desired consistency. Keep well covered in refrigerator no longer than 2 days.

NOTE:

This is not the tastiest soup, but it is full of healing goodness. My mother-in-love, Barbara Griswold, would bring me her version, using spicy tomatoes, adding more cabbage and green peppers, and she did not put it through the food mill. All of the vegetables were chopped and stewed, and I actually preferred her version to my own. Hippocrates, the father of modern day medicine, actually used a recipe very close to this for his patients; it is an important part of the Gerson protocol and can be found on page 102 of the *Gerson Therapy Handbook* mentioned above.

7:30 pm FRESH JUICE:

Fresh carrot juice - see rpage 90.

8:00 pm LIVER DETOX:

Same as page 90.

Helpful Resources

Books and Videos

During my own quest for answers, I was fortunate to come across some very impactful books and videos. Most all of the videos can be found on YouTube or Netflix. Find out the truths for yourself. Be an informed patient and look at the evidence closely. Study those patients who have done well, and healed strong. Look at the evidence. Understand the science behind it. Don't take anyone's word at face value. Seek wisdom and gain understanding.

Books and Videos/Audio CD

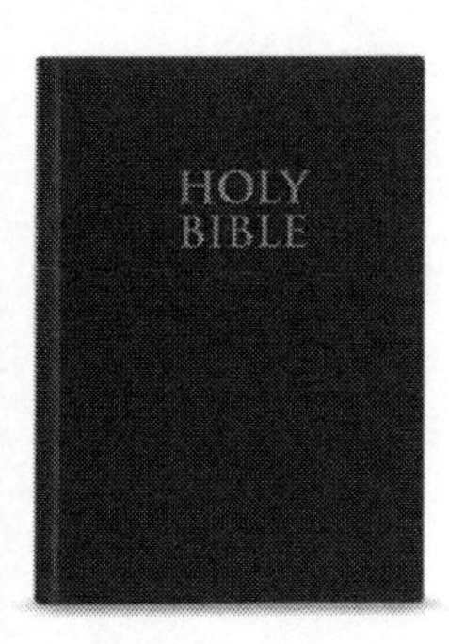

The Bible

I searched scriptures for promises from God regarding healing. I listened to them daily for several months, and then used my time of detox to continue to search scriptures. It has been the most important aspect of my healing journey. The Bible is the living word of Creator God.

An audio CD or MP3 that can be downloaded and is packed full of healing scriptures and beautiful music can be found at: https://larryhutton.org/product/heavens-health-food/

Heaven's Health Food by Larry S. Hutton

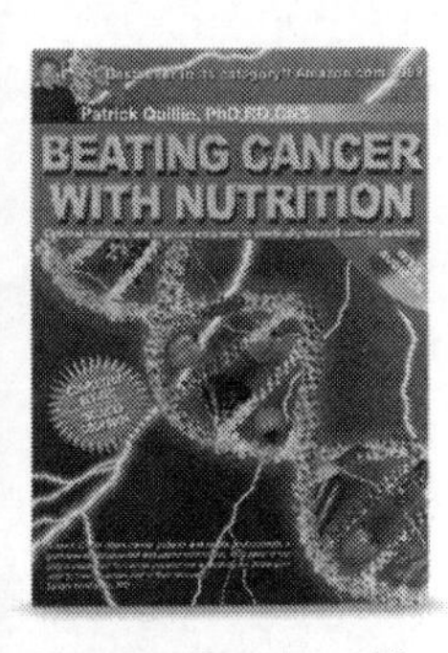

Beating Cancer with Nutrition
by Dr. Patrick Quillin

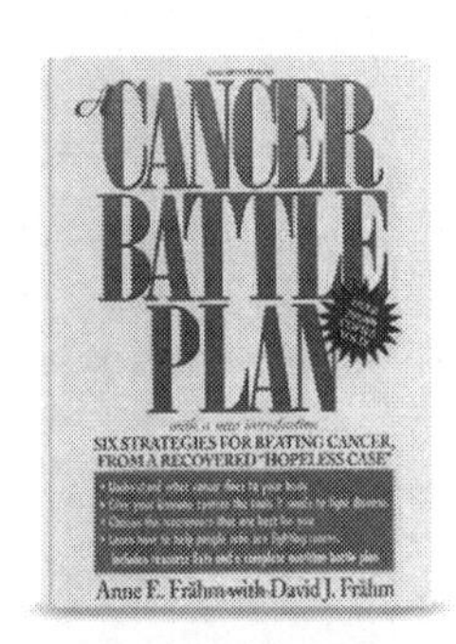

A Cancer Battle Plan
by Anne Frahm

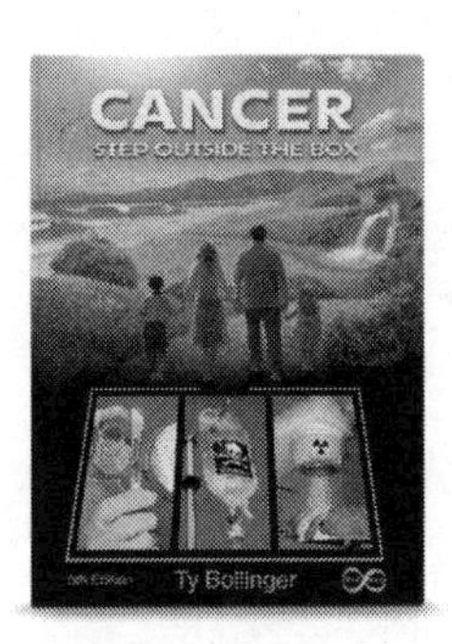

Cancer: Step Outside the Box
by Ty Bollinger

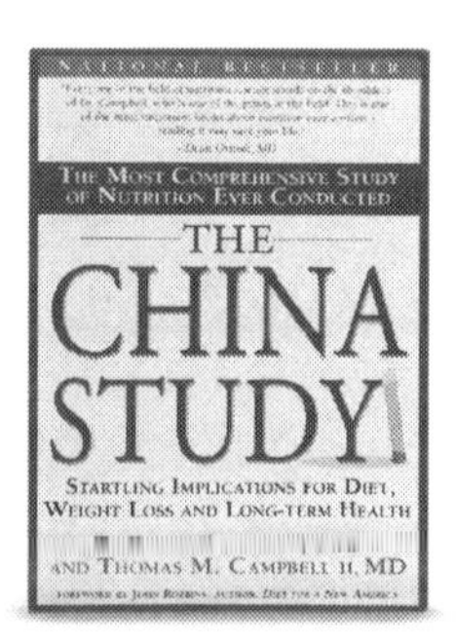

The China Study
by T. Colin Campbell

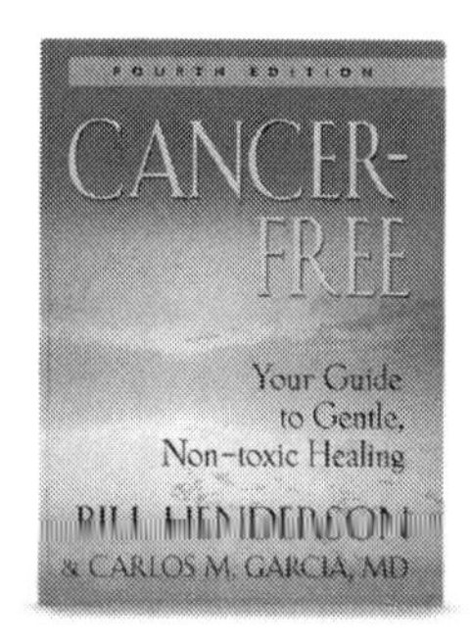

Gentle Non-Toxic Healing
by Bill Henderson

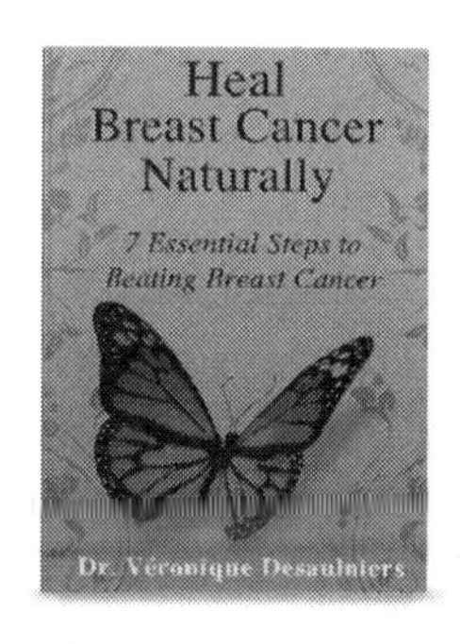

Heal Breast Cancer Naturally
by Dr. Veronique Desaulniers

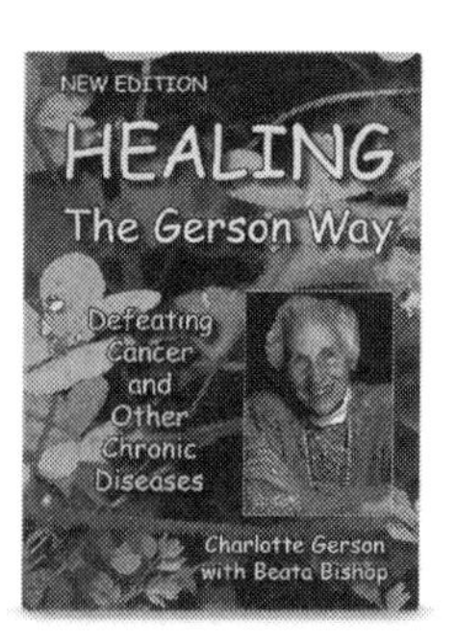

Healing the Gerson Way
by Charlotte Gerson

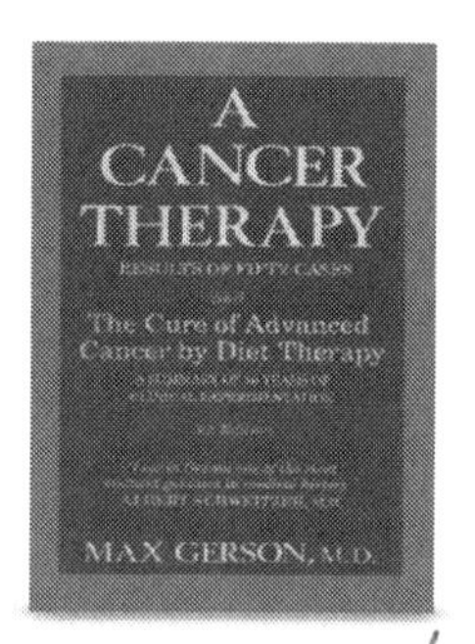

A Cancer Therapy: Results of Fifty Cases
by Dr. Max Gerson

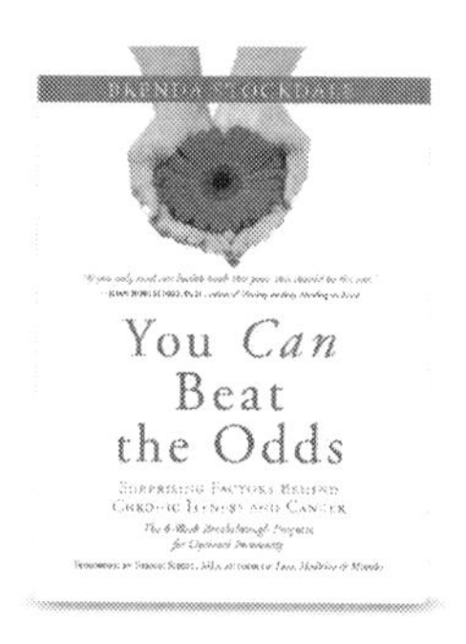

You Can Beat the Odds
by Brenda Stockdale

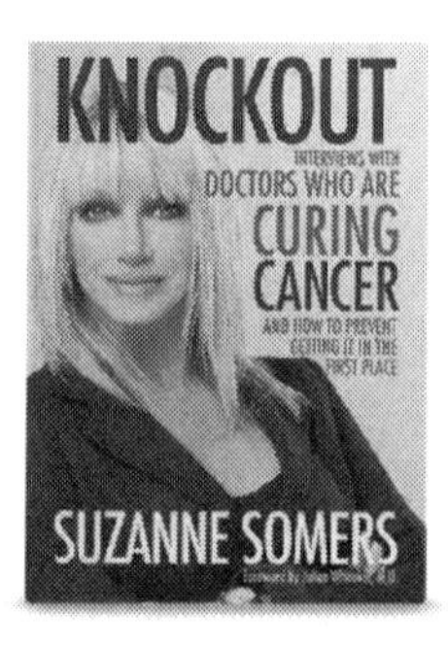

Knockout
by Suzanne Somers

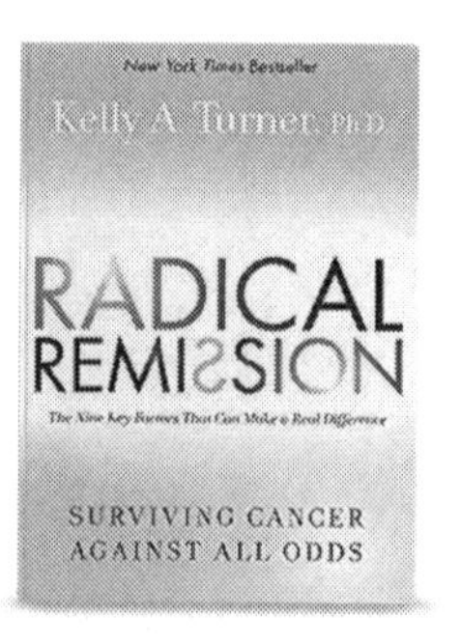

Radical Remission
by Dr. Kelly Turner

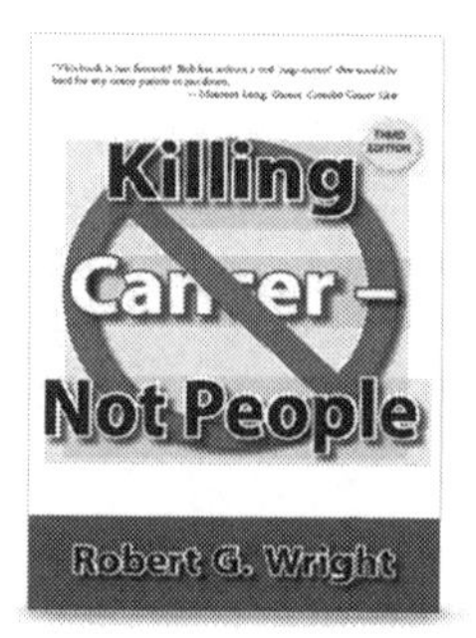

Killing Cancer Not People
by Bob Wright

Recommended Video Series Available Online:

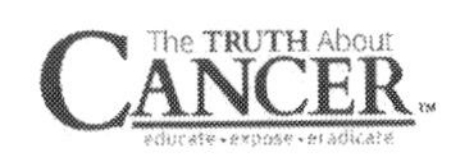

The Truth About Cancer Series (Quest for the Cures): https://go2.thetruthaboutcancer.com/global-quest/replay/?a_aid=56034d-b58e51d&a_bid=8ec340aa

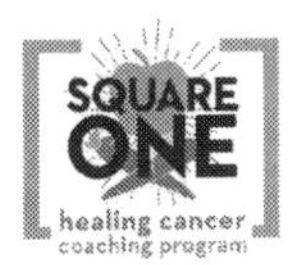

Square One (A Holistic Survivors Step by Step Approach): https://sn188.infusionsoft.com/go/go/HealingStrong

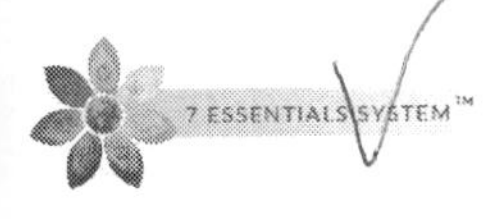

7 Essentials System™ (A complete and step-by-step educational program to live vibrant health). https://jk232.isrefer.com/go/NFBCA/HealingStrong/

Additional Videos

- *The Burzynski Movie: Cancer is Serious Business*
- *Fat, Sick and Nearly Dead (on Netflix)*
- *Forks Over Knives (on Netflix)*
- *The Gerson Miracle (on Netflix)*
- *A Global Quest*
  (Complete docu-series by The Truth About Cancer)
- *Simply Raw for 30 Days*
- *Super Juice Me*

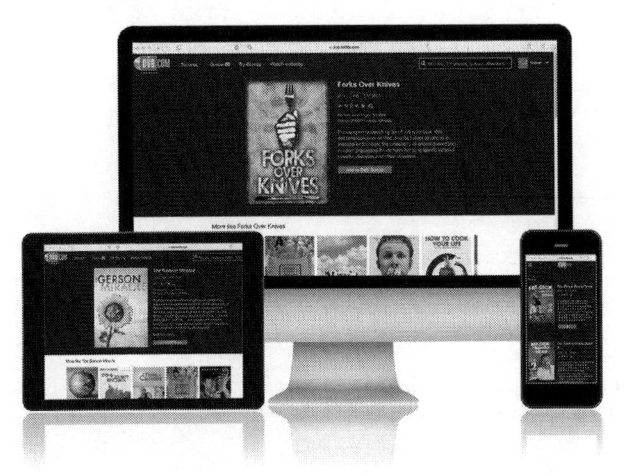

Websites/Non-profit Organizations

There are many good websites you can go to for researching cancer data, holistic treatments, testimonials, recipes and other information to support you in your healing journey. There are also some supportive non-profit organizations that can provide additional information and help you along the way.

Websites

healingstrong.org

cancercompassalternateroute.com (best testimonials)

anticancermom.com

alkalinesisters.com (recipes)

believebig.org

breastcancerconqueror.com

breastcancerchoices.com

cancertruth.net

cancertutor.com

chrisbeatcancer.com

ewg.org (product safety)

healthnutnews.com

juiceladycherie.com

kriscarr.com (recipes)

mercola.com

naturalnews.com

organicfacts.net

robertscottbell.com

thetruthaboutcancer.com

Non-profit Organizations

HealingStrong
www.healingstrong.org

Cancer Crackdown
www.cancercrackdown.org
Helps with supplements and offers a coaching program.

P4 Foundation
www.p4foundation.org
For children with cancer.

American Anti-Cancer Institute
americanaci.org

Nicholas Gonzalez Foundation
dr-gonzalez.com

Center for Advancement in Cancer Education
beatcancer.org

Believe Big
believebig.org

Annie Appleseed Project
annieappleseedproject.org

Independent Cancer Research Foundation
cancertutor.com

Recommended Clinics and Physicians

Finding the right physician can be valuable in your journey. I personally watched the Gerson DVDs and read books and articles. I encourage folks to find a wellness advocate (whether it is a naturopath, physician, health coach) or someone else who will support your journey. Keep in mind, they are not the ones who will heal you. YOU are responsible for your health. You spend a fraction of the time with a practitioner and the majority away from him or her. YOU have to find a protocol that suits you best and COMMIT, making adjustments along the way.

If you can't afford a doctor (insurance usually doesn't cover a natural approach to healing), go to www.cancercrackdown.org or Beatcancer.org, which offer support and coaching. There are also clinics that can help you, nutritionists and holistic providers who may be in your area. When you connect with a local HealingStrong™ group (www.healingstrong.org/groups), most leaders will have a local resource lists that they or their group has compiled, and share them with their participants.

Physicians and Clinics in the United States

Center for Advanced Medicine
Cornelius, NC
Rashid Bhuttar, DO
drbuttar.com

Namaste Health Center
Durango, CO
Michele Hemingway, MD
namastehealthcenter.com

Cancer Center for Healing
Irvine, CA
Leigh Erin Connealy, MD
cancercenterforhealing.com

Dr. Douglas Wichman
Atlanta, GA
advancedrejuvenationinstitute.com

Dr. Kevin Conners
Minneapolis, MN
connersclinic.com

Linda Isaacs, MD
NYC
www.drlindai.com

An Oasis of Healing
Mesa, AZ
Thomas Lodi, MD
anoasisofhealing.com

Dr. Daniel Nuzum
Nampa and Meridian, ID
Drnuzum.com

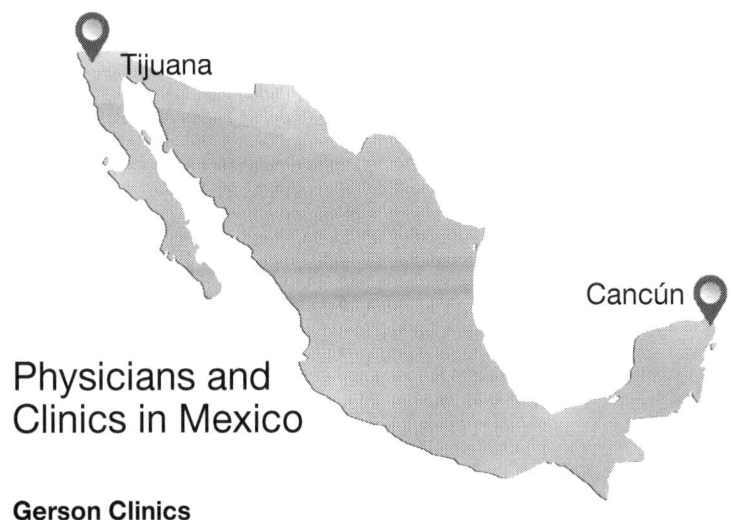

Physicians and Clinics in Mexico

Gerson Clinics
gerson.org/gerpress/gerson-clinic-mexico
gerson.org/gerpress/gerson-health-centre

Northern Baja Healing Center
(Gerson Therapy, plus adjunct therapies)
Tijuana, Mexico
gersontreatment.com

CHIPSA
(Gerson Therapy, plus adjunct therapies)
Tijuana, Mexico
chipsahospital.org

Hoxsey Biomedical Center
Tijuana, Mexico
hoxseybiomedical.com

Hope 4 Cancer Institute
Tijuana & Cancun, Mexico
Dr. Tony Jiminez
www.hope4cancer.com

Clinica MTC
Dra. Mei Hung Lee Lai
clinicamtc.com.mx

Jump-Start Days/Week-Long Retreats

Healing Diva Retreat
breastcancerconqueror.com

Hallelujah Acres
hacres.com

Living Foods Institute
livingfoodsinstitute.com

Hippocrates Institute
hippocratesinst.org

Cherie Calbom
Juicing /Raw Foods Retreats
juiceladycherie.com

NOTES

Thank you God! Amen

Made in the USA
Columbia, SC
26 September 2018